The North Star Diet
And
Weight Management
Program

By

Gregory T. Mucha, M.D.

Notice:

This book is intended as a reference volume only, not as a medical text. The information given here is designed to help adults 18 years and older make informed decisions about their health. It is not intended as a substitute for any treatment. If you suspect that you have a medical problem, I urge you to seek medical help.

Mention of specific companies, organizations, or authorities in this book does not imply endorsement by the publisher, nor does mention of specific companies, organizations, or authorities imply that they endorse this book.

Internet addresses given in this book were accurate at the time it went to press.

www.thenorthstardiet.com

Printed in the United States of America
North Star Diet Inc

ISBN 0-9772287-0-3

Introduction

The North Star Diet and Weight Management Program is the result of my desire to educate individuals about safe and effective weight loss and weight maintenance. I was frustrated by many popular diet texts, the Atkins Diet, South Beach Diet, and Zone Diet, which have failed to address many of the components of safe and effective weight loss and weight maintenance. The information contained in this book has been distributed to numerous patients in my practice with highly successful results. My text allows individuals to lose weight by utilizing customized meal plans based on the nutritional guidelines of the Institute of Medicine. The Institute of Medicine is the governmental institution which makes recommendations for the entire United States based on a critical review of all available medical and nutritional information. My book differs greatly from other resources because I provide calorie-specific meal plans and exercise routines which allow an individual to achieve weight loss and then maintain a stable weight.

Contents

Strength Training Day # 2

Strength Training Day # 3

Alternate exercise regimen

Adequate sleep

Daily vitamins/supplements

Stress reduction

Limiting fast food consumption

Why am I not achieving my weight-loss goals utilizing the North Star Diet and Weight Management Program?

How do you determine your weight-maintenance caloric requirements?

Are prescription weight-loss medications safe and effective?

Does weight-loss surgery cure obesity?

Fiber chart

Resting energy calculator

Caloric diary sample page

Acknowledgements:

Text edited by L. J. Miller.

Thank you:

   Miller family: Barrie, Lindsay, Lois, Patrick, and Robert.

   Mucha family: Carol, Tara, and Theodore.

Notice:

Part One: Understanding the North Star Diet and Weight Management Program

Why use the North Star Diet and Weight Management Program?

The North Star Diet and Weight Management Program was created to provide individuals with a straightforward and no-nonsense program to lose weight and to achieve their physical fitness goals while enjoying satisfying foods. In my medical practice I have utilized the diet and exercise regimens contained in this book to help my patients achieve optimal weight loss and physical fitness goals. The North Star Diet employs the guidelines established by the Institute of Medicine and enables an individual to lose weight by consuming nutritious foods specifically chosen for their ability to promote satiety, or feelings of fullness. The weight management portion of the book is concerned with sustaining weight loss achieved with the North Star Diet.

The North Star Diet and Weight Management Program is unique because it allows individuals to achieve their goals by simply employing the 5 points of the North Star Diet. Each point will be explained more fully in Part Two. The points are:

1) Consume food every 2-3 hours during the day.
2) Decrease daily fat consumption by half.
3) Increase carbohydrate consumption in the form of fiber by 7- 9 grams per week, to achieve the optimal minimal daily amounts of 25 grams for adult females, and 40 grams for adult males.
4) Obtain adequate daily protein.
5) Perform daily exercise.

The program is both comprehensive and flexible, with a variety of options available for each user. Many individuals have achieved success by simply following the 5 point outline of the North Star Diet and Weight Management Program. Others, who enjoy more structure, will achieve success by following the gender-specific meal plans and rules in Part Three and Part Four. A step-wise, less-structured plan called the progression version is available in Part Five.

I do not accept failure so I have also included a custom-designed weight-loss program (in Part Eight) for those who do not achieve their desired weight loss with the regular diet. Once individuals have achieved their weight-loss goals they are encouraged to sustain their weight loss by employing the weight-management calculator found in Part Eight.

The North Star Diet and Weight Management Program derives its name from the state in which I reside, Minnesota, also called the North Star State. Two of the essential nutrients emphasized in this program, dietary fiber and soy protein, are both produced in abundance in Minnesota. The

North Star Diet is not a fad diet. It utilizes the nutritional recommendations of the most recent report of the Institute of Medicine. The Institute of Medicine is the governmental institution which makes recommendations for the entire United States based on a critical review of all available medical and nutritional information.

The dietary composition of the North Star Diet and Weight Management Program has been purposefully conceived to make it appealing, effective, and sustainable. It is built around eating fruits, vegetables, and lean, low-fat protein in the form of chicken, turkey, seafood, lean beef, pork, and soy. Appealing snacks are encouraged throughout the day.

How the North Star Diet and Weight Management Program is different from other diets and a review of popular diets.

A variety of diets and programs have recently gained prominence with the public. I will briefly discuss some of the merits and shortcomings of each diet/plan and explain why the North Star Diet and Weight Management System is more nutritionally sound and effective.

Weight Watchers as an organization relies upon group support and a dietary system in which each food has been given a point value. Attendees at meetings give and receive invaluable encouragement for their weight-loss efforts. Unfortunately, many individuals abuse the point system and do not eat a balanced diet with sufficient levels of carbohydrate in the form of dietary fiber as well as adequate protein to achieve satiety, or the feeling of fullness. Many individuals choose to spend their allotted points on high-carbohydrate, high-fat selections, such as ice cream, candy, and deep-fried foods. In contrast, the North Star Diet encourages a nutritionally sound diet, high in fiber and with adequate amounts of protein, in a dietary format that is also appealing in variety and flavor. This is a low-calorie diet that is satisfying, that is it promotes satiety, and it improves health. The dietary composition of the North Star Diet lowers your risk of heart attacks, strokes, and, potentially, your risks for developing numerous types of cancers.

The South Beach Diet, Zone Diet, and Atkins Diet are largely based on the belief that low- or very-low-carbohydrate diets produce greater weight loss than traditional diets. Rigorous long-term studies have recently been published which reveal greater weight loss with lower-calorie, but not reduced-carbohydrate content diets. North Star is different from South Beach, Zone, and Atkins because it promotes carbohydrate consumption, especially in the form of high-fiber carbs.

A popular concept called the glycemic index is a system for classifying carbohydrate-containing foods according to how fast they raise blood glucose levels inside the body. The South Beach and Atkins diets discourage the consumption of corn, baked potatoes, peas, and other foods which have an elevated glycemic index number. I am not concerned with the glycemic content of carbohydrates but instead with their fiber content so I encourage the consumption of foods with a high fiber content irrespective of the glycemic index number of the foods. Thus, the North Star Diet encourages the consumption of various moderate- to high-glycemic foods, such as corn, baked potatoes, peas, watermelon, and wild rice because they contain high levels of fiber.

The North Star Diet is full of appealing fruits and vegetables and lean protein in the form of broiled meats, fish and/or soy. It is a diet which will improve your cardiovascular health and reduce your risk of stroke and heart attack. The two key essential components of the North Star Diet are carbohydrates high in dietary fiber, and adequate amounts of low-fat (lean) protein, in the form of chicken, fish, turkey, lean beef, pork, and/or soy. The benefits of fiber and lean protein are reported in numerous scientific publications and by experts in the field of nutrition. Fiber and lean protein assist in weight loss, weight maintenance, reduction of heart disease, stroke, and possibly various types of cancer.

The North Star Diet and Weight Management Program also differs from the currently popular diets in that the weight-maintenance portion of the book acts as a personal trainer. This section provides clear illustrations and descriptions of suggested exercises to help you get started on a physical fitness regimen and begin to enjoy its benefits regardless of your age or physical limitations. The North Star Diet and Weight Management Program is unique because it incorporates the most recent and accurate scientifically proven nutritional and exercise advice.

Testimonials

"I have lost 20 lbs a month by following the diet, 80 lbs total since starting the diet. I am not hungry and my energy has improved."

Peter R

"The recipes are great. I shared them with my friend who is a chef, he also finds them appealing."

John M

"My goal was to lose 10 lbs. I was able to lose the weight in 5 weeks with no feelings of hunger by following the meal plans."

Lisa R

"I did not qualify for weight loss surgery. The surgeon said I was too high of a risk. I was sent to meet with Dr. Mucha and I have been following the North Star Diet and have lost 70 pounds in 3 months."

Paula S

"I never thought I could lose weight by eating three meals and snacks a day. I am not hungry at all."

Peter T

"The fiber in the diet is easy to consume, and Dr. Mucha was right, I am not hungry if I obtain enough fiber in my diet."

John R

"I enjoyed reading the book. It answered many questions I had concerning weight loss and current popular diets."

Robin R

"The North Star dietary rules are easy to follow, and make sense."

Janice Q

"The lunch wraps are easy to make, and the selection is great."

Robert F

"The weight maintenance portion is easy to follow; I particularly enjoy the exercise review guides."

June S

"The daily exercises have been easy to complete and follow."

Beth R

Part Two:
The Five Points of The North Star Diet

1) Consume meals and/or snacks approximately every 2-3 hours throughout the day.

2) Decrease your daily fat consumption by half.

3) Increase daily carbohydrate consumption in the form of fiber by 7-9 grams per week until a total of 25 to 40 grams per day is achieved.

4) Obtain adequate daily protein.

5) Perform daily exercise.

NORTH STAR POINT # 1
Consume meals and/or snacks approximately every 2-3 hours throughout the day.

Consuming smaller meals more frequently promotes weight loss. The traditional diet in the US has been primarily dependent on two large meals, at noon and in the evening. Breakfast is often skipped or neglected. A study in the American Journal of Epidemiology revealed that people who eat small meals many times a day are less likely to be obese than those who eat fewer meals. Those consuming food four or more times daily, generally three meals and one or two snacks, were the least likely to be obese. People who regularly skipped breakfast were far more likely to be obese. The study also found that people eating breakfast or dinner away from home were more likely to be overweight. This is most likely secondary to larger portions, and the higher fat content of restaurant or fast food meals.

The consumption of smaller meals throughout the day is beneficial because it can increase an individual's metabolism and promote fat loss. Researchers in England have demonstrated that regularity of meals promotes increased energy expenditure. In their study nine healthy women were asked to continue with their normal diet for 14 days in one of two patterns:

1) Six small meals per day, eaten at regular intervals.
2) Three to nine meals per day, eaten at irregular intervals and varied at random times throughout the 2-week period.

After two weeks, the women resumed their previous eating patterns for two weeks, and then switched to the other eating pattern for two weeks. Results indicate that irregular meal frequency led to a lower after-meal metabolic rate as compared with regular meal frequency.

The North Star Diet incorporates meals and snacks throughout the day with the following guidelines:

A) I encourage the consumption of three meals a day and two snacks. (Examples of daily menus can be found in Parts Three and Four.)

B) Snacks should consist of foods that promote satiety, or feelings of fullness. These are foods that satisfy hunger and are high in fiber or protein. Preferred snack choices are:
  - banana
  - apple
  - pear
  - strawberries, 2 cups (no sugar added)
  - blueberries, 1 1/2 cups (no sugar added)
  - raspberries, 2 cups (no sugar added)
  - low-calorie yogurt (100 calories)
  - soy nuts, 1 oz. or 100 calories total (varies based on brand and preparation)
  - soy chips, 1 oz. (I recommend Revival brand soy chips)

Three to four times a week, if you like, you may substitute any food you desire (100 to 200 calories depending upon your meal plan, Part Three and Part Four), for example a part-skim mozzarella cheese stick, or 1 oz dark chocolate (100 calories).

C) I recommend that no food should be consumed during the 3-4 hours prior to going to bed. Consumption of food close to bedtime is more likely to cause weight gain. This is because during periods of sleep your metabolism decreases and the excess food calories may be stored as fat. If you need to eat closer to bedtime select one of the above snack choices, as they will satisfy your hunger more effectively than many other foods high in fat and sugar.

NORTH STAR POINT # 2
Decrease your daily fat consumption by half.

Fat is a source of energy for the body and aids in the absorption of essential vitamins. Unfortunately, the average daily adult consumption of fat in the United States often exceeds 40-60% of total caloric intake. High-fat diets are also very high in calories. Essentially, fat contains twice the energy as the equivalent amount of protein or carbohydrate. Fat, along with protein and carbohydrates, supplies calories to the body, at nine calories/gram for fat compared to four calories/gram for carbohydrates and protein. Therefore I recommend, as a guide, that you decrease the fat content of your diet by about half in an **effort** to reduce your calories. All of the North Star Diet meal plans (Part Three and Part Four) are calculated to contain 30% or less total fat, including 8-10% saturated fat.

The relatively high calorie content of fat makes it very important to keep the quality high while lowering the quantity. Because of this we need to think of fat in terms of healthy and non-healthy fats. The non-healthy fats are saturated fat and trans fats . These are the fats that give fat its bad reputation because they are responsible for elevating cholesterol levels, which in turn promotes heart disease and stroke. Saturated fats are found in animal products such as butter, cheese, whole milk, ice cream, cream, and fatty meats such as certain red meats and various pork products. Trans fatty acids or trans fats form when vegetable oil is hardened, a process known as hydrogenation. The resulting product can raise the "bad" cholesterol or LDL. Trans fats are found in fried foods, commercial baked goods (donuts, cookies, crackers), processed foods, and margarines. Saturated fats and trans fats provide no beneficial role in preventing chronic disease. No study has ever revealed any associated health benefit with the consumption of either. Thus the panel from the National Academies Institute of Medicine recommends limiting consumption of total fat to 20-35% of total calories and saturated fat to 10% or less, and attempting to avoid all food products containing trans fats .

Healthy fats are the unsaturated fats . Two types of unsaturated fats exist - monounsaturated fats and polyunsaturated fatty acids . Monounsaturated fats reduce blood cholesterol levels and lower the risk of heart disease when they replace saturated and trans fats in the diet. Polyunsaturated fats supply essential fatty acids, or EFAs. The body does not make these fatty acids and must get EFAs from food. EFAs are vital to the human brain and central nervous system. They also produce hormone-like substances that help regulate blood pressure, blood clotting, and the immune system.

Unsaturated fat sources consist of liquid vegetable oils. Peanut, canola, and olive oil are monounsaturated oils, which lower an individual's cholesterol. Coconut, palm, and palm kernel oils, often used in restaurants, are not monounsaturated oils, and can elevate an individual's cholesterol level. One must always remember that, although monounsaturated oils are beneficial in that they lower cholesterol, they are still very high in calories, and if consumed in large amounts can promote weight gain.

Polyunsaturated fatty acids, also present in fat, reduce blood cholesterol levels and lower the risk of heart disease when they replace saturated fats in the diet. Two types of polyunsaturated fats, Omega-3 fatty acids (alpha-linolenic acid) and Omega-6 fatty acids (linoleic acid), are known as essential fatty acids . Because the body cannot synthesize these fatty acids they must be obtained from food. Omega-3 fatty acids can be obtained from cold-water fish, including tuna, salmon, and mackerel, and from dark green leafy vegetables and flaxseed oil. Omega-3 fatty acids have been found to be beneficial to the heart. Positive effects include anti-inflammatory and anti-blood clotting actions, lowering cholesterol and triglyceride levels, and reducing blood pressure. These fatty acids may also reduce the risks and symptoms for other disorders including diabetes, stroke, some cancers, and dementia.

Omega-6 is another essential fatty acid. It is found in sunflower, corn, sesame, and soybean oils. It appears that in the United States consumption of Omega-6 has increased dramatically compared to Omega-3 fatty acids . Excess intake of Omega-6 fatty acids can cause increased water retention, elevated blood pressure, and the potential for an increased risk of blood clots. In theory we should reduce our consumption of Omega-6 fatty acids and increase our consumption of Omega-3 fatty acids. Omega-6 and Omega-3 essential fatty acids are best consumed in a ratio of about 3:1, or three Omega-6 to one Omega-3.

NORTH STAR POINT # 3

Increase daily carbohydrate consumption in the form of fiber by 7-9 grams a week until a total of 25-38 grams per day is achieved.

Several low-carbohydrate diets have gained great popularity in the last couple of years. The Atkins, Zone, and South Beach diets are all based on the belief that carbohydrates promote elevated levels of insulin which subsequently causes weight gain. Numerous recent long-term studies have revealed that the total number of calories consumed is a more important factor. Carbohydrates in the form of fruits and vegetables do not promote weight gain unless eaten in excess.

It is best to think of carbohydrates as consisting of available and unavailable carbohydrates. Available carbohydrates are those that are reduced by enzymatic action in the human gastrointestinal system to simple sugars (lactose, glucose, and fructose) that are then absorbed by the small intestine. These simple sugars are found in such foods as fruit, syrups, grain products and milk. Enzymes are protein complexes that facilitate chemical manipulations within organisms. Enzymes do not break down unavailable carbohydrates. Dietary fiber is the most common form of unavailable carbohydrate that individuals consume in their diet. Carbohydrates are an excellent source of nutrients as long as they are in a form consisting of both available carbohydrates (simple sugars) and unavailable carbohydrates (fiber).

Fruits and vegetables that contain large amounts of fiber have many benefits:

1) Fiber promotes satiety, or the feeling of fullness.

Numerous studies have demonstrated that a higher-fiber diet produces satiety in the short term. In one study, obese diabetic men weighing approximately 250 pounds were fed a high-fiber diet providing 32 grams of fiber during an 800-calorie diet for 10 days. They then changed to a low-fiber diet providing 8 grams of dietary fiber per 800 calories for 10 days. On the higher-fiber diet, the feeling of satiety was greater at each time point during the day than on the lower-fiber diet. Numerous other studies have also revealed that dietary fiber intake decreases calorie consumption and promotes satiety.

A simple example I use to illustrate the satiety power of fiber is the relationship between apples and a candy bar. Most candy bars contain 200-300 calories, and 0 grams of fiber. Everyone can easily consume a candy bar. However, the caloric equivalent of a candy bar is 3-4 large apples. Very few individuals can consume 4 apples at one time. Apples simply provide a greater degree of satiety because they contain 4g of fiber in each apple versus the candy bar's 0 grams.

The benefits of high fiber intake for weight maintenance have not been established in long-term studies. These studies are often difficult to complete because subjects realize when their diets contain more fiber. Therefore, it is difficult to have a blinded group in a study; that is, a group that is unaware that their food is being manipulated. Food manipulation or pharmaceutical drugs are only considered effective if a study can reveal an improved outcome compared to a placebo – a non-manipulated diet, or a sugar pill in pharmaceutical trials. Nevertheless, I am absolutely convinced, through personal experience with patients, that the intake of high-fiber foods contributes to successful weight maintenance.

2) High-fiber diets lower heart disease risk.

Current fiber guidelines from the Food and Nutrition Board are based on studies that show an increased risk for heart disease when diets low in fiber are consumed. Diets high in fiber reduce blood sugar levels. Any reduction in blood sugar levels helps prevent the development of diabetes. Diabetes is associated with an increased risk of cardio-vascular disease.

3) High-fiber diets improve blood sugar control.

High-fiber diets slow and decrease the absorption of sugar and fat in the intestine. They lower blood glucose values, and decrease cholesterol and triglyceride levels. High-fiber diets are capable of diminishing the need for insulin or oral hypoglycemic agents utilized in the treatment of type II diabetes.

High-fiber diets also promote weight loss, which acts synergistically to improve diabetes, and to lower cholesterol, which can decrease an individual's risk for heart disease and stroke.

4) Fiber reduces cancer risk.

Higher-fiber diets most likely decrease colon cancer, however more long-term studies need to be completed. The most recent long-term evaluation in the United States, the Nurses' Health Study, found no difference in the incidence of colorectal cancer between those who consumed a low-fiber diet and those who ate a high-fiber diet. Nevertheless, many other studies contradict this one study. Future long-term investigation in the United States and other Western countries will be needed to help clarify the role of fiber as a colon cancer protective agent. It is a well-known fact that the incidence of colon cancer is significantly lower in cultures where people consume diets high in fiber.

Essential dietary fiber facts: Q and A.

Q. How much fiber should I obtain in my diet?

A. The National Academies Institute of Medicine recommends that the total daily intake of fiber for adults 50 years and younger is 38 grams for men and 25 grams for women. Men and women over age 50 should consume a minimum of 30 grams, for men, and 21 grams, for women, secondary to decreased consumption of food. Nevertheless, there are individuals who consume greater than 60g of fiber a day to better control their type II diabetes and are able to tolerate the high-fiber diets well, with dramatic improvements in their blood glucose control.

Q. What foods contain fiber?

A. The majority of individuals in the United States are uncertain how to increase the fiber content of their diet. The average adult in the Unites States obtains only 6-10 grams of fiber daily. An alphabetic listing of common foods and their fiber content can be found in Part Nine. All of the meal plans provided in the North Star Diet achieve the goal of 30 or more grams of fiber a day.

An essential component of the North Star Diet is the daily consumption of a high-fiber breakfast. All breakfasts should contain a minimum of 8 grams of fiber. High-fiber breakfasts can only be achieved by consuming high-fiber cereals or wraps made with tortillas containing at least 10 grams of fiber and filled with eggs or, preferably, egg substitutes. A list of excellent high-fiber cereals, oatmeal and tortilla/wraps follows.

CEREAL	PORTION	CALORIES	FIBER (content)
General Mills Fiber One	1/2 cup	59	14 g
General Mills Fiber One Honey Clusters	1 1/4 cup	170	14 g
Kellogg's Bran Buds	1/3 cup	80	11 g
Kellogg's All-Bran	1/2 cup	80	10 g
Post or Nabisco			
100% Bran	1/3 cup	80	9 g
Post Raisin Bran	1 cup	190	8 g
Kashi Good Friends	3/4 cup	90	8 g
Kashi Lean Crunch	1 cup	190	8 g
OATMEAL			
Quaker Weight Control	1 serving	160	6 g
TORTILLAS			
Cruz whole-wheat	large 8"	130	11 g
La tortilla factory	large 8"	80	14 g
Mission low carb	6" size	110	11 g

Q. How should I increase the fiber content of my diet?

A. The fiber content in an individual's daily diet should be increased slowly by no more than 7-10 grams per week. The North Star Diet meal plans gradually increase the fiber content of the diet by 7-10 grams a week, with a goal of 30 grams daily by the third week. You should be aware that if you attempt to increase your fiber consumption from the average of 6-10 grams a day to the optimal 30 grams a day all at once, you would most likely experience bloating, gas, and diarrhea.

Q. Should I increase the fiber in my diet with fiber pills or powder?

A. I do not recommend the use of fiber in the form of psyllium, which is the main form of fiber found in fiber-bulking powders such as Metamucil, Fibercon, and Citrucel. Each serving generally contains 3 grams of fiber. In comparison, an average size apple contains 4 grams of fiber and is both nutritious and satisfying. The fiber goals recommended by the Institute of Medicine, 25-38 grams, are very difficult to reach using supplemental fiber pills or powders.

The second reason I do not recommend fiber in the form of psyllium seeds is that it can produce constipation if it is not consumed with generous amounts of water. Psyllium has tremendous water-absorbing capacity, more than other types of fiber. This means that if individuals do not consume large amounts of fluid, at least ten 8-ounce glasses of water a day, or two 8-ounce glasses of water with each meal and two snacks, they could develop constipation.

Q. Do I need to increase the fluid I consume on a higher-fiber diet?

A. I encourage all individuals to consume approximately one 8-ounce glass of water 10 times a day, or two 8-ounce glasses with each of their three meals and two snacks. Individuals may choose to substitute some of the daily water intake with diet soda (pop in the Midwest), or green tea. Recent studies revealed that two cups of green tea increase thermogenesis, the process by which the body burns calories. Subjects who consumed two cups of green tea burned approximately 70 more calories a day. We also recommend that individuals eliminate regular soda pop from their diet and minimize fruit juice consumption. Fruit juice should be replaced with whole fruit, which is high in nutrition but low in total calories.

The purpose of increasing your fluid intake is threefold. One, it prevents dehydration. Two, it promotes satiety. Three, it prevents the development of constipation on a high-fiber diet. This is because your intestine does not absorb a large percentage of fiber. Since fiber has a high water-absorbing capacity it can promote constipation if an individual is not adequately hydrated.

NORTH STAR POINT # 4
Obtain adequate daily protein.

It is essential that all individuals obtain adequate levels of protein in their diet. The Institute of Medicine recommends that adults should obtain 10-35% of their total calories from protein, or approximately .8 grams per kg of body weight for adults. The following chart illustrates the range of appropriate protein consumption based on a variety of caloric intakes.

APPROPRIATE DAILY PROTEIN INTAKE

Caloric Intake	Protein (Grams) 10% of Total Calories	Protein (Grams) 35% of Total Calories	Protein (Ounces) 10% of Total Calories	Protein (Ounces) 35% of Total Calories
1200 Calories	30 g	105 g	1 oz	3.5
1400 Calories	35 g	123 g	1.2 oz	3.75
1600 Calories	40 g	140 g	1.4 oz	4.9
1800 Calories	45 g	158 g	1.6 oz	5.6
2000 Calories	50 g	175 g	1.76 oz	6.17

The above chart reveals that the minimum amount of daily protein (10% of total calories) required in a 1200-calorie diet is 30 grams, which is the equivalent of 4 ounces of ground meat, or 6.3 ounces of tofu. The maximum amount of protein (35% of total calories) required in a 1200-calorie diet is 105 grams, or the amount found in 12-13 ounces of lean meat or 24 ounces of tofu. Three ounces of protein approximates the volumetric space occupied by a deck of playing cards.

Adequate levels of protein are required to maintain a healthy lifestyle and are essential components of any lower-calorie diet or maintenance diet. There is convincing evidence that higher-protein diets are beneficial for three reasons. Higher-protein diets increase satiety, or feelings of fullness. They are also believed to increase thermogenesis, or metabolism, compared to diets low in protein.

Adequate levels of protein during a low-calorie diet also help prevent muscle wasting or loss due to malnutrition. Often, individuals who follow lower-calorie diets fail to consume enough protein. If an individual takes in less than 10 % of their total daily caloric intake in the form of protein, they can develop protein deficiency and loss of muscle mass, as the human body will break down the skeletal muscle mass to provide energy for the body. The only individuals who should be concerned about limiting their protein intake, potentially below the Institute of Medicine recommendations of 10-35% of their total calories, are individuals with decreased kidney function. The majority of adults do not suffer from impairment of kidney function, but if your health care provider has told that your kidney function is less than optimal, confer with him or her for dietary protein guidelines.

Protein should be consumed in the form of lean broiled meats, fish, chicken, soy, or whey protein powder. Examples of lean protein are listed in the following chart, including type, serving size in ounces, and actual ounces and grams of protein provided by the serving size.

PROTEIN CONTENT OF VARIOUS MEATS, TOFU, AND WHEY POWDER

Type of Protein	Amount	Protein Content (in ounces)	Protein Content (in grams)
Grilled Chicken (skinless/ no skin)	4 oz	1.15 oz	32.8 g
Grilled Lean Beef (fat trimmed)	4 oz	1.15-1.34 oz	32-38 g
Grilled Fish	4 oz	.95 oz	27 g
Roasted Turkey (without the skin)	4 oz	1.2 oz	33.9 g
Lean Pork (white meat)	4 oz	1.12 oz	32 g
Tofu	4 oz	.63 oz	18 g
Whey Powder	4 oz	3.2 oz	92.3 g

An excellent source of protein often neglected in western diets is soy. Numerous studies have revealed the benefits of soy. Soy protein is believed to promote satiety, lower the risk of heart disease, and decrease menopausal symptoms. Soy protein may also help prevent bone loss, endometrial cancer and prostate cancer.

Many of the beneficial properties of soy are secondary to their estrogenic activity. Soy contains compounds known as isoflavones that are capable of estrogen-like effects. Estrogens are signaling molecules that exert their effects by binding to estrogen receptors within cells. Estrogen receptors are present in numerous tissues other than those associated with reproduction, including bones, liver, heart, and brain. Soy isoflavones bind to estrogen receptors in some tissues and block the effects of estrogen in other tissues. A considerable amount of scientific research is currently being conducted concerning soy isoflavones. The interest is due to their potential tissue-specific, anti-estrogenic, and estrogenic effects. The anti-estrogenic effects in reproductive tissue could help reduce the risk of hormone-associated cancers (breast, uterine, and prostate), while the estrogenic effects in other tissues could help maintain bone density and improve cholesterol levels.

We encourage individuals to consume soy products on a daily basis, in the form of soymilk with high-fiber cereal or oatmeal, and in the form of soy nuts and soy pasta chips.

Numerous myths exist concerning soy products. The most common is that soy products promote hypothyroidism, or low thyroid levels. High intakes of soy isoflavones do not appear to increase the risk of hypothyroidism, as long as dietary iodine consumption is adequate. Fortunately, iodine is found in abundance in the United States, as iodine is bound to almost all forms of salt sold in the United States. Numerous studies have been completed with both premenopausal and postmenopausal women in which high intakes of soy isoflavones resulted in no clinically significant alterations in thyroid hormone levels.

The only individuals I do not recommend consuming soy are adolescent males, pregnant females, and breast cancer survivors. Soy protein is most likely not damaging in these individuals, however no long-term, well-controlled studies have ever been completed which exclude adverse consequences. The potential adverse consequences of excess soy consumption in adolescent males could be the development of breast tissue. Contrary to popular belief excess breast tissue in males is a reasonably common finding, 36%, with or without soy consumption.

Excess isoflavone intake during pregnancy is most likely safe. However, the safety of isoflavone supplements during pregnancy has not been established. I do not recommend high intakes of soy for breast cancer survivors. The effects of high intakes of soy isoflavones in breast cancer survivors is an area of considerable debate among scientists and clinicians. Some animal studies have found that soy isoflavones can stimulate the growth of estrogen- receptor-positive breast cancer cells. These are cells which multiply at a faster rate when stimulated by estrogens. A few human studies suggest that increased consumption of soy isoflavones can have estrogenic effects in human breast tissue. Many experts believe that women with a history of breast cancer, particularly estrogen-positive breast cancer, should not increase their consumption of phytoestrogens, including soy isoflavones.

NORTH STAR POINT # 5   Perform daily exercise.

The importance of daily exercise cannot be over-emphasized. It is essential that individuals complete daily activity to maintain health. No medications or supplements will ever replace or provide the benefits achieved by daily exercise.

Benefits of daily exercise:
* Increases physical fitness.
* Helps build and maintain healthy bones, muscle, and joints.
* Builds endurance and muscular strength.
* Helps manage weight.
* Lowers risk factors for cardiovascular disease, colon cancer, breast cancer, type II diabetes.
* Helps control blood pressure.
* Promotes psychological well-being and self-esteem.
* Reduces feelings of depression and anxiety.
* Prevents or delays onset of Alzheimer's disease.

The current national guidelines are to achieve 60-90 minutes of moderate activity on a daily basis. Moderate activity is equivalent to the amount of exertion experienced during a moderate walk in which you would still be able to speak to a partner comfortably. Vigorous activity is the equivalent of a light jog. I recommend that you begin with mild or moderate exercise for 10-20 minutes a day, gradually increasing the time weekly, with an ultimate daily goal of 60-90 minutes of moderate activity or 30 minutes of vigorous activity per day. Studies have shown that several 10-minute bouts of exercise are as effective as 30 consecutive minutes for weight maintenance and cardiovascular fitness. The current national guidelines of 60-90 minutes of moderate activity or 30 minutes of vigorous activity each day are based on numerous studies which reveal that individuals can maintain a stable weight, long-term, with that level of exercise.

Individuals using the North Star Weight Management Plan may participate in any form of exercise they find interesting or enjoyable. Popular and effective forms of exercise include walking, cycling, running, aerobics, and swimming. The exercise promoting the greatest benefit for both losing excess weight and then maintaining the new level is strength training. Strength training, if completed properly, allows one to increase muscle mass and maintain aerobic fitness. Women over the age of 20 lose, on average, half a pound of muscle per year, for a total of five pounds per decade. If a female remains at the same weight during a decade with little daily activity, she will often have replaced muscle with fat. This loss of muscle may be a primary reason that women often gain 15 pounds of fat each decade. Because each pound of muscle burns 35-40 calories a day, a female could lose an additional half pound of fat in six weeks just by adding a pound of muscle through strength training, without any dietary changes.

The accumulation of lean muscle mass is beneficial for multiple reasons: including improving strength and balance, maintaining bone mass, and increasing metabolic rate. The best method for accumulating muscle mass is strength training. Strength training, if done properly, with 30-60 seconds between sets, allows individuals to elevate their heart rate to a level equivalent to a brisk walk. It provides an individual with a maximum number of benefits: accumulation of muscle mass, an elevated metabolism, and improved cardiovascular fitness. A large portion of this book is dedicated to teaching individuals to incorporate strength training into their exercise regimen in a safe, effective, and inexpensive manner. The fitness directions appear in Part Six.

Part Three:
Customized Meal Plans

We recommend the following calorie-restrictive meal plans based on your starting weight and gender. As you lose weight continue to select the weight appropriate dietary plan. The meal plans are calculated to allow for safe, effective weight loss and contain optimal amounts of fiber, protein, fat, and other essential nutrients.

FEMALES:

Weight in lbs	Dietary Plan
≤250 lbs	1200 Calorie
≥250 ≤300 lbs	1400 Calorie
≥300 lbs	1600 Calorie

MALES:

Weight in lbs	Dietary Plan
≤250 lbs	1400 Calorie
≥250 ≤300 lbs	1600 Calorie
≥300 lbs	1800 Calorie

1200 CALORIE DIET

Calorie Distribution in 1200 Calorie Diet

Breakfast	250 Calories
Mid-Morning Snack	100 Calories
Lunch	375 Calories
Mid-Afternoon Snack	100 Calories
Dinner	375 Calories

Rules for the North Star Diet

1) Eat breakfast within 20 minutes after waking in the morning. Failure to eat a timely breakfast will decrease your fat-burning capacity, or metabolism. Breakfast choices consist of any high-fiber cereal with non-fat milk fortified with vitamin D and calcium or, preferably, non-fat soy milk fortified with vitamin D and calcium. High-fiber cereals should contain at least 8 grams of fiber in each serving. Recommended high-fiber cereals:

CEREAL	PORTION	CALORIES	FIBER (content)
General Mills Fiber One	1/2 cup	59	14 g
General Mills Fiber One Honey Clusters**	1 1/4 cup	170	14 g
Kellogg's Bran Buds	1/3 cup	80	11 g
Kellogg's All-Bran	1/2 cup	80	10 g
Post or Nabisco			
100% Bran	1/3 cup	80	9 g
Post Raisin Bran	1 cup	190	8 g
Kashi Good Friends	3/4 cup	90	8 g
Kashi Lean Crunch	1 cup	190	8 g
OATMEAL			
Quaker Weight Control	1 serving	160	8 g
TORTILLAS			
Cruz whole-wheat	large 8"	130	11 g
La tortilla factory	large 8"	80	14 g
Mission low carb	6" size	110	11 g

2) Consume mid-morning snacks and mid-afternoon snacks. Both snacks may consist of one (1200 calorie diet) or two (all other diets) of the following choices: banana; apple; pear; 2 cups strawberries (no sugar added); 1.5 cups blueberries (no sugar added); 2 cups raspberries (no sugar added); low-calorie yogurt (100 calories); 1 oz of soy nuts (100 calories total, varies based on brand and preparation); 1 oz soy chips (I recommend Revival brand soy chips). Failure to eat timely mid-morning and mid-afternoon snacks will decrease your fat-burning capacity, or metabolism. Three to four times a week you may substitute any food you desire(100 to 200 calories depending upon meal plan), for example one or two part-skim mozzarella cheese stick(s) or 1-2 oz of chocolate (100-200 calories).

Rules for the North Star Diet, cont'd

3) Consume 2 liters of fluid a day (approximately 80 ounces). Eighty ounces of fluid is the equivalent of 8 ounces of water per hour for ten hours a day, or two 8-ounce glasses of water with each meal and snack. You may substitute diet soda pop or tea with meals if desired but no fruit juice or regular pop is allowed.

4) Consumption of two cups of green tea, one tea bag per cup, will promote 70 calories of weight loss on a daily basis. A personal favorite is Tazo Zen brand of green tea.

5) Consume dinner 3-4 hours prior to bed time. If you eat closer to bedtime there is an increased chance the food will be stored and converted into fat while you sleep. If you are still hungry after dinner, you may consume an apple, pear or banana or 1 ounce of lean, grilled protein, e.g. turkey, ham, beef, or fish.

6) The meal plans are to be used as guides. Most individuals only eat 7-10 different foods in a given week. If you like certain wraps or dinners and not others, consume those you enjoy the most. I only ask that starting in the second week of the North Star Diet you begin utilizing a whole-wheat wrap/tortilla. (See lunch alternative if you desire to use bread as an alternative). Whole-wheat wraps can often contain as much as 10–14 g of fiber per serving. They are easy to make. Combine fillings in the center of the tortilla and roll up. I recommend the following whole-wheat tortilla/wraps: Cruz brand whole-wheat tortilla (10 grams of dietary fiber per serving); La Tortilla Factory whole-wheat, low-carb/low-fat tortillas (large size, 14 grams of fiber); and Carb Down flat bread (14 grams of fiber).

7) Consume daily: a multi-vitamin; 1200 mg of calcium carbonate; 1000 I.U. vitamin D; and 1000-3000 mg of fish oil.

** Personal Favorite

Measurement Conversions

Do not fear the measurements in the following calorie-specific diets. You could weigh each item as described. However, I approximate all food quantities based on the volume of a deck of playing cards.

3 ounces (oz) = the fluid volume of a deck of playing cards.

1 cup = 8 fluid ounces = 2.5 fluid equivalents of a deck of playing cards.

1 ounce (oz) = the fluid equivalent of one-third of a deck of playing cards.

1/2 ounce (oz) = 1 tablespoon (tbsp) = the fluid equivalent of 1/6 of a deck of playing cards.

1200 CALORIES

Week 1 * Day 1

BREAKFAST: One cup of cereal (see cereal choices) and one cup soymilk or low fat or skim milk.

MID-MORNING SNACK: Snacks may consist of one of the following choices: banana; apple; pear; 2 cups strawberries (no sugar added); 1.5 cups blueberries (no sugar added); 2 cups raspberries (no sugar added); low-calorie yogurt (100 calories); 1 oz of soy nuts (100 calories total, varies based on brand and preparation); 1 oz soy chips (I recommend Revival brand soy chips. Three to four times a week, if desired, you may substitute any 100-calorie food you desire, for example a part-skim mozzarella cheese stick or 1 oz of chocolate (100 calories).

LUNCH: Mediterranean Wrap
      8" tortilla wrap
      4 oz turkey, roasted or sliced, skinless white meat
      4 lettuce leaves
      2 oz cucumber strips
      1 tsp red pepper flakes
      1 oz Feta cheese
      2 tsp fat-free red wine vinegar

MID-AFTERNOON SNACK: Same as mid-morning snack.

DINNER: Crispy Baked Chicken, with rice and vegetable.

Family size (4 servings)	Single serving
2-2.5 lbs boneless, skinless chicken breasts	6 oz boneless, skinless chicken breast
1 cup skim milk	1/4 cup skim milk
1 cup cornflake crumbs	1/4 cup cornflake crumbs
1 tsp rosemary	1 pinch rosemary
1 tsp fresh ground black pepper	1 pinch fresh ground black pepper
Pam cooking oil spray or olive oil spray	Pam cooking oil spray or olive oil spray

Preheat oven to 350 degrees. Cover a baking dish with foil and spray lightly with cooking oil spray. Rinse chicken and pat dry. Set aside. Pour milk into a shallow bowl. Combine cornflake crumbs, rosemary, and pepper in another shallow bowl. Dip chicken first into milk and then into crumb mixture. Allow to stand briefly so coating will adhere. Arrange chicken in prepared pan so pieces do not touch. Bake 40 minutes or until done. Crumbs will form a crisp "skin".

Serve with 3/4 cup of cooked wild or brown rice and 1 cup of any of the following steamed vegetables: asparagus, broccoli, eggplant, green beans, kale, snow pea pods, or spinach.

1200 CALORIES

Week 1 * Day 2

BREAKFAST: One cup of cereal (see cereal choices) and one cup soy milk or low-fat or skim milk.

MID-MORNING SNACK: Snacks may consist of one of the following choices: banana; apple; pear; 2 cups strawberries (no sugar added); 1.5 cups blueberries (no sugar added); 2 cups raspberries (no sugar added); low-calorie yogurt (100 calories); 1 oz of soy nuts (100 calories total, varies based on brand and preparation); 1 oz soy chips (I recommend Revival brand soy chips. Three to four times a week, if desired, you may substitute any 100-calorie food you desire, for example a part-skim Mozzarella cheese stick or 1 oz of chocolate (100 calories).

LUNCH: Beef Taquito Wrap
   8" tortilla wrap
   4 oz round steak, trimmed
   1 oz mozzarella low-fat cheese
   2 tsp salsa

MID-AFTERNOON SNACK: Same as mid-morning snack.

DINNER: Scallops Oriental, with rice and vegetable.

Family size (4 servings)	Single serving
cooking oil spray (preferably olive oil)	cooking oil spray (preferably olive oil)
1 lb fresh or frozen scallops	4 oz fresh or frozen scallops
1/8 cup honey	2 tsp honey
1/8 cup mustard	2 tsp mustard
1/2 tsp curry powder	pinch curry powder
1/2 tsp lemon juice	1/8 tsp lemon juice

Preheat broiler. Lightly spray baking pan with cooking spray. Rinse scallops and drain. Place in a baking pan. In a saucepan, combine remaining ingredients. Brush scallops with sauce. Broil 4 inches from heat for 5-8 minutes or until browned.

Serve with 3/4 cup of cooked wild or brown rice and 1 cup of any of the following steamed vegetables: asparagus, broccoli, eggplant, green beans, kale, snow pea pods, or spinach.

1200 CALORIES

Week 1 * Day 3

BREAKFAST: One cup of cereal (see cereal choices) and one cup soy milk or low-fat or skim milk.

MID-MORNING SNACK: Snacks may consist of one of the following choices: banana; apple; pear; 2 cups strawberries (no sugar added); 1.5 cups blueberries (no sugar added); 2 cups raspberries (no sugar added); low-calorie yogurt (100 calories); 1 oz of soy nuts (100 calories total, varies based on brand and preparation); 1 oz soy chips (I recommend Revival brand soy chips. Three to four times a week, if desired, you may substitute any 100-calorie food you desire, for example a part-skim mozzarella cheese stick or 1 oz of chocolate (100 calories).

Lunch: Tuna Mayo Wrap
    8" tortilla wrap
    1.5 oz low-fat mayonnaise
    6 oz tuna
    1/4 rib celery

MID-AFTERNOON SNACK: Same as mid-morning snack.

DINNER: Tomato, Mushroom, and Jack Cheese Omelet, with vegetable and baked potato.

Single serving
    Cooking oil spray (olive oil preferable)
    2 eggs or egg substitute equivalent
    1/4 cup seeded, chopped tomato
    1/2 oz shredded, low-fat Monterey jack cheese
    1/4 cup mushrooms
    1 tsp chopped cilantro or parsley
    Hot pepper sauce (optional)

Spray skillet with cooking oil, or use non-stick frying pan. Place pan over medium high heat. In a small bowl, place eggs or egg substitute. Beat and pour mixture into pan. Stir eggs in a circular motion. Do not scrape bottom of pan. When the omelet is almost cooked, add fillings. Fold omelet over with a fork while holding the pan at 45-degree angle. Roll omelet onto plate and serve.

Serve with 1 medium (7 oz) baked potato with 1 tsp soft canola margarine, and 1 cup of any of the following steamed vegetables: asparagus, broccoli, eggplant, green beans, kale, snow pea pods, or spinach.

1200 CALORIES

Week 1 * Day 4

BREAKFAST: One cup of cereal (see cereal choices) and one cup soy milk or low-fat or skim milk.

MID-MORNING SNACK: Snacks may consist of one of the following choices: banana; apple; pear; 2 cups strawberries (no sugar added); 1.5 cups blueberries (no sugar added); 2 cups raspberries (no sugar added); low-calorie yogurt (100 calories); 1 oz of soy nuts (100 calories total, varies based on brand and preparation); 1 oz soy chips (I recommend Revival brand soy chips. Three to four times a week, if desired, you may substitute any 100-calorie food you desire, for example a part-skim mozzarella cheese stick or 1 oz of chocolate (100 calories).

LUNCH: Beef Wrap
   8" tortilla wrap
   4 oz round steak, trimmed, broiled
   1/2 cup of raw or broiled mushrooms
   2 tsp Worcestershire sauce
   1 tsp soy sauce

MID-AFTERNOON SNACK: Same as mid-morning snack.

DINNER: Mustard-Crusted Pork, with rice and vegetable.

Serving for two
   2 tsp soy or tofu flour (available at most health food stores)
   1 tsp mustard powder
   1/2 tsp pepper
   1/4 cup olive oil
   1 lb boneless, center cut pork chops, cut against the grain into 3" strips, about 3/8 " thick

Single serving
   2 tsp soy or tofu flour (available at most health food stores)
   1 tsp mustard powder
   1/2 tsp pepper
   1/4 cup olive oil
   8 oz boneless, center-cut pork chops, cut against the grain into 3" strips, about 3/8 " thick

Combine the flour, mustard powder, and pepper in a bowl and mix well. Dust the pork with the flour mixture. Heat 2 tbs oil over medium heat until hot but not smoking. Add half the pork and brown for five minutes on each side, or until cooked through. Repeat with the remaining pork. Sprinkle with seasoning. Remove from heat and serve immediately.

Serve with 3/4 cup of cooked wild or brown rice and 1 cup of any of the following steamed vegetables: asparagus, broccoli, eggplant, green beans, kale, snow pea pods, or spinach.

1200 CALORIES

Week 1 * Day 5

BREAKFAST: One cup of cereal (see cereal choices) and one cup soy milk or low-fat or skim milk.

MID-MORNING SNACK: Snacks may consist of one of the following choices: banana; apple; pear; 2 cups strawberries (no sugar added); 1.5 cups blueberries (no sugar added); 2 cups raspberries (no sugar added); low-calorie yogurt (100 calories); 1 oz of soy nuts (100 calories total, varies based on brand and preparation); 1 oz soy chips (I recommend Revival brand soy chips. Three to four times a week, if desired, you may substitute any 100-calorie food you desire, for example a part-skim mozzarella cheese stick or 1 oz of chocolate (100 calories).

LUNCH: Turkey Vegetable Wrap
   8" tortilla wrap
   4 oz turkey, roasted or sliced, skinless white meat
   1 oz corn, canned in water
   1 oz red pepper
   1 oz green onion
   2 tsp fat-free, light ranch dressing

MID-AFTERNOON SNACK: Same as mid-morning snack.

DINNER: Fish Fillets with Asparagus, with rice and vegetable.

Family size (serves four)	Single serving
Cooking oil spray (preferably olive oil)	Cooking oil spray (preferably olive oil)
4 - 5 oz mild, white fish fillets (Haddock, cod, etc.)	5 oz mild, white fish fillet (Haddock, cod, etc.)
1/2 tsp ground black pepper	1/4 tsp ground black pepper
2 tbsp unsalted butter	1 tbsp unsalted butter
12 stalks cooked asparagus	4 stalks cooked asparagus
1/3 cup tangy sour cream	1/3 cup tangy sour cream
1/3 cup plain low-fat yogurt	1/3 cup plain low-fat yogurt
2 tsp minced chives	1 tsp minced chives
2 tsp horseradish	1 tsp horseradish
1 egg white	1 egg white
2 tsp chopped parsley	1 tsp chopped parsley

Preheat broiler. Lightly spray broiler pan with cooking spray. Rinse fish and pat dry. Season fish with pepper and lemon juice and brush with margarine. Place on broiler pan and broil about 8 minutes or until fish almost flakes. Remove from oven and top each filet with 3 stalks of asparagus. In a small bowl, combine sour cream, yogurt, chives, horseradish, and dill weed. In another bowl, beat egg whites until stiff peaks form; fold into sour cream mixture. Spread mixture over each fillet to cover fish and asparagus. Return to broiler and broil 1-2 minutes, or until golden brown. Sprinkle with parsley.

Serve with 3/4 cup of cooked wild or brown rice and 1 cup of any of the following steamed vegetables: asparagus, broccoli, eggplant, green beans, kale, snow pea pods, or spinach.

1200 CALORIES

Week 1 * Day 6

BREAKFAST: One cup of cereal (see cereal choices) and one cup soy milk or low-fat or skim milk.

MID-MORNING SNACK: Snacks may consist of one of the following choices: banana; apple; pear; 2 cups strawberries (no sugar added); 1.5 cups blueberries (no sugar added); 2 cups raspberries (no sugar added); low-calorie yogurt (100 calories); 1 oz of soy nuts (100 calories total, varies based on brand and preparation); 1 oz soy chips (I recommend Revival brand soy chips. Three to four times a week, if desired, you may substitute any 100-calorie food you desire, for example a part-skim mozzarella cheese stick or 1 oz of chocolate (100 calories).

LUNCH: California Chicken Wrap
   8" tortilla wrap
   3 oz grilled white chicken
   2 tsp guacamole
   3 tomato slices
   3 lettuce leaves
   1 tsp bacon bits

MID-AFTERNOON SNACK: Same as mid-morning snack.

DINNER: Feta Burgers, with rice and steamed vegetable.

Family size (serves 4)	Single serving
Cooking oil spray, preferably olive oil	Cooking oil spray, preferably olive oil
1 lb ground sirloin or ground round	4 oz ground sirloin or ground round
1/4 cup crumbled feta cheese	1 oz feta cheese
1/4 cup finely-chopped black olives	1 oz finely-chopped black olives
1/2 tsp salt	pinch of salt
1/2 tsp. pepper	pepper to taste

Heat pan sprayed with cooking spray. Mix remaining ingredients and shape into four patties (one for single serving). Sauté patties at medium high heat for 5 minutes on each side or to desired doneness.

Serve with 3/4 cup of cooked wild or brown rice and 1 cup of any of the following steamed vegetables: asparagus, broccoli, eggplant, green beans, kale, snow pea pods, or spinach.

1200 CALORIES

Week 1 * Day 7

BREAKFAST: One cup of cereal (see cereal choices) and one cup soy milk or low-fator skim milk.

MID-MORNING SNACK: Snacks may consist of one of the following choices: banana; apple; pear; 2 cups strawberries (no sugar added); 1.5 cups blueberries (no sugar added); 2 cups raspberries (no sugar added); low-calorie yogurt (100 calories); 1 oz of soy nuts (100 calories total, varies based on brand and preparation); 1 oz soy chips (I recommend Revival brand soy chips. Three to four times a week, if desired, you may substitute any 100-calorie food you desire, for example a part-skim mozzarella cheese stick or 1 oz of chocolate (100 calories).

LUNCH: Ham Club Wrap
  8" tortilla wrap
  4 oz ham
  3 tomato slices
  3 lettuce leaves
  1 tsp bacon bits
  1 tsp light Italian dressing
  1 oz low-fat mozzarella cheese

MID-AFTERNOON SNACK: Same as mid-morning snack.

DINNER: Lemon Baked Chicken, with rice and steamed vegetable.

Family size (serves 4)	Single serving
Olive oil cooking spray	Olive oil cooking spray
2 tsp fresh lemon juice	1 tsp fresh lemon juice
2 tsp low-fat margarine or **safflower** oil	1 tsp low-fat margarine or **safflower** oil
1 clove garlic, crushed	1 / 4 clove garlic, crushed
1/2 tsp fresh ground black pepper	1/ 8 tsp fresh ground black pepper
2–2.5 lbs of boneless, skinless chicken breast	6 oz boneless, skinless chicken breast

Preheat oven to 350 degrees. Lightly spray a baking pan or a shallow casserole dish with cooking spray. In a small bowl, combine lemon juice, oil, garlic and pepper. Set aside. Rinse chicken and pat dry. Arrange chicken in prepared pan or dish. Pour lemon mixture over chicken pieces. Cover and bake 40 minutes or until tender, basting occasionally. Uncover and bake 10 minutes longer to allow chicken to brown.

Serve with 3/4 cup of cooked wild or brown rice and 1 cup of any of the following steamed vegetables: asparagus, broccoli, eggplant, green beans, kale, snow pea pods, or spinach.

1200 CALORIES

Week 2 * Day 1

BREAKFAST: One cup of cereal (see cereal choices) and one cup soy milk or low-fat or skim milk.

MID-MORNING SNACK: Snacks may consist of one of the following choices: banana; apple; pear; 2 cups strawberries (no sugar added); 1.5 cups blueberries (no sugar added); 2 cups raspberries (no sugar added); low-calorie yogurt (100 calories); 1 oz of soy nuts (100 calories total, varies based on brand and preparation); 1 oz soy chips (I recommend Revival brand soy chips.Three to four times a week, if desired, you may substitute any 100-calorie food you desire, for example a part-skim mozzarella cheese stick or 1 oz of chocolate (100 calories).

LUNCH: Chicken with Zucchini and Roasted Pepper Wrap
   8" whole-wheat tortilla wrap
   4 oz broiled white chicken meat
   3-4 oz zucchini
   2 oz pickled sweet peppers
   1 oz part-skim, reduced-fat mozzarella cheese

MID-AFTERNOON SNACK: Same as mid-morning snack.

DINNER: Pineapple and Shrimp, with rice and vegetable.

Family size (Serves 4)	Single serving
1 clove garlic	1 tsp garlic powder or 1/4 clove of garlic
2 tsp canola margarine	2 tsp canola margarine
1/4 cup honey	1 oz honey
1 tbsp sweet chili sauce	1 tsp sweet chili sauce
1 tbsp soy sauce	1 tsp of soy sauce
1 whole pineapple, or 20 oz canned in water or light syrup	6 oz fresh pineapple, or 6 oz canned in water or light syrup
2 lbs shrimp, fresh or frozen, peeled and de-veined	6 oz shrimp, fresh or frozen, peeled and de-veined

Combine first five ingredients in a bowl. Brush shrimp with the mixture. Grill at high temperature for 5 minutes. Add pineapple.

Serve with 3/4 cup of cooked wild or brown rice and 1 cup of any of the following steamed vegetables: asparagus, broccoli, eggplant, green beans, kale, snow pea pods, or spinach.

1200 CALORIES

Week 2 * Day 2

BREAKFAST: One cup of cereal (see cereal choices) and one cup soy milk or low-fat or skim milk.

MID-MORNING SNACK: Snacks may consist of one of the following choices: banana; apple; pear; 2 cups strawberries (no sugar added); 1.5 cups blueberries (no sugar added); 2 cups raspberries (no sugar added); low-calorie yogurt (100 calories); 1 oz of soy nuts (100 calories total, varies based on brand and preparation); 1 oz soy chips (I recommend Revival brand soy chips. Three to four times a week, if desired, you may substitute any 100-calorie food you desire, for example a part-skim mozzarella cheese stick or 1 oz of chocolate (100 calories).

LUNCH: Santa Fe Steak Burrito
   8" whole wheat tortilla wrap
   2 oz steak
   1 oz corn
   3 oz black beans
   1 tsp sour cream
   3 lettuce leaves
   3 tomato slices
   1 oz low-fat mozzarella cheese
   2 tsp salsa

MID-AFTERNOON SNACK: Same as mid-morning snack.

DINNER: Turkey Burgers, with wild rice and vegetable.

Family size (serves 4)	Single serving
1 lb ground turkey (90% lean), raw, thawed	4 oz ground turkey (90% lean), raw, thawed
1/4 cup onions, or powdered onion flakes	1 oz onions, or powdered onion flakes
2 tbsp green peppers	2 tsp green peppers
1 tbsp Worcestershire Sauce	1 tsp Worcestershire sauce
2 tbsp ketchup	1 tsp ketchup
1/4 tsp black pepper	1/8 tsp black pepper
lettuce leaves	lettuce leaves
tomato slices	tomato slices
4 whole-wheat pita pockets	1 whole-wheat pita pocket

Form ground turkey and seasonings into patties. Grill or broil for 5 minutes per side, or until done. Top patties with lettuce and tomato and place in pita pocket.

Serve with 4 oz (1/2 cup) of cooked brown or wild rice and 1 cup of any of the following steamed vegetables: asparagus, broccoli, eggplant, green beans, kale, snow pea pods, or spinach.

1200 CALORIES

Week 2 *Day 3

BREAKFAST: One cup of cereal (see cereal choices) and one cup soy milk or low-fator skim milk.

MID-MORNING SNACK: Snacks may consist of one of the following choices: banana; apple; pear; 2 cups strawberries (no sugar added); 1.5 cups blueberries (no sugar added); 2 cups raspberries (no sugar added); low-calorie yogurt (100 calories); 1 oz of soy nuts (100 calories total, varies based on brand and preparation); 1 oz soy chips (I recommend Revival brand soy chips. Three to four times a week, if desired, you may substitute any 100-calorie food you desire, for example a part-skim mozzarella cheese stick or 1 oz of chocolate (100 calories).

LUNCH: Tasty Turkey Wrap
  8" whole-wheat tortilla wrap
  onion powder to taste
  4 oz turkey
  2 tsp olives
  1 oz mozzarella low-fat cheese
  2 tsp fat-free mayo
  3 lettuce leaves
  1 tsp mustard
  3 slices tomato

MID-AFTERNOON SNACK: Same as mid-morning snack.

DINNER: Chicken with Mushrooms, with baked potato and vegetable.

Family size (serves 4)	Single serving
4 - 6 oz chicken breasts, skinless	6 oz chicken breast, skinless
20 oz button mushrooms	5 oz button mushrooms
1/2 tsp pepper	1 pinch of pepper
1 garlic clove	1/4 garlic clove
2 tbsp olive oil	1 tbsp olive oil
juice of half a lemon	juice of 1/4 lemon
1 cup dry white wine	1/2 cup dry white wine
pinch of dried hot red pepper flakes	pinch of dried hot red pepper flakes

Grill chicken, set aside. Heat oil in a heavy skillet over medium heat. Add the garlic, lemon juice, wine, pepper, and red pepper flakes. Bring to a boil. Lower heat and add mushrooms. Simmer and stir frequently for 5–6 minutes. Add pre-grilled chicken.

Serve with 1 medium (7 oz) baked potato, with 1 tsp soft canola margarine, and 1 cup of any of the following steamed vegetables: asparagus, broccoli, eggplant, green beans, kale, snow pea pods, or spinach.

1200 CALORIES

Week 2 * Day 4

BREAKFAST: One cup of cereal (see cereal choices) and one cup soy milk or low-fat or skim milk.

MID-MORNING SNACK: Snacks may consist of one of the following choices: banana; apple; pear; 2 cups strawberries (no sugar added); 1.5 cups blueberries (no sugar added); 2 cups raspberries (no sugar added); low-calorie yogurt (100 calories); 1 oz of soy nuts (100 calories total, varies based on brand and preparation); 1 oz soy chips (I recommend Revival brand soy chips. Three to four times a week, if desired, you may substitute any 100-calorie food you desire, for example a part-skim mozzarella cheese stick or 1 oz of chocolate (100 calories).

LUNCH: Greek Wrap
   8" whole-wheat tortilla wrap
   4 oz grilled chicken breast, no skin
   1 oz feta cheese (reduced-fat)
   4 lettuce leaves
   2-3 tomato slices
   2 tsp low-calorie vinaigrette dressing

MID-AFTERNOON SNACK: Same as mid-morning snack.

DINNER: Pork with Green Chile and Cheese, and rice and vegetable.

Family size (serves 4)
   1.5 lbs boneless, center-cut loin pork chops or sirloin pork steaks (fat removed)
   2 tbsp olive oil
   1/2 cup green chili salsa
   3/4 cup low-fat cheese, shredded (feta, Muenster, cheddar, or mozzarella)

Single serving
   6 oz boneless, center-cut loin pork chops or sirloin pork steaks (fat removed)
   1 tsp olive oil
   2 oz green chili salsa
   2 oz low-fat cheese, shredded (feta, Muenster, cheddar, or mozzarella)

Heat oil in pan over medium heat until hot but not smoking. Add pork to pan and brown for 3-5 minutes. Turn heat to low, add 1/2 cup water, and cover pan. Cook for 20-25 minutes or until water is nearly evaporated. Pour salsa over pork, covering evenly. Sprinkle with shredded cheese, cover and cook for additional 3 to 5 minutes or until salsa is heated and cheese is melted.

Serve immediately with 6 oz (3/4 cup) of cooked brown or wild rice and 1 cup of any of the following steamed vegetables: asparagus, broccoli, eggplant, green beans, kale, snow pea pods, or spinach.

1200 CALORIES

Week 2 * Day 5

BREAKFAST: One cup of cereal (see cereal choices) and one cup soy milk or low-fat or skim milk.

MID-MORNING SNACK: Snacks may consist of one of the following choices: banana; apple; pear; 2 cups strawberries (no sugar added); 1.5 cups blueberries (no sugar added); 2 cups raspberries (no sugar added); low-calorie yogurt (100 calories); 1 oz of soy nuts (100 calories total, varies based on brand and preparation); 1 oz soy chips (I recommend Revival brand soy chips. Three to four times a week, if desired, you may substitute any 100-calorie food you desire, for example a part-skim mozzarella cheese stick or 1 oz of chocolate (100 calories).

LUNCH: Bean and Cheese Burrito
   8" whole-wheat tortilla wrap
   2 oz reduced-fat Cheddar cheese
   5 oz black beans
   3 lettuce leaves

Heat, if desired, in microwave or toaster oven.

MID-AFTERNOON SNACK: Same as mid-morning snack.

DINNER: Tandoori Chicken, with rice and vegetable.

Family Size (serves 4)
   4 - 6 oz chicken breasts, skinless
   3 tsp tandoori spice mix
   1 tsp fresh ginger, grated
   1 1/2 cups plain, non-fat yogurt

Single serving
   1 - 6 oz chicken breast, skinless
   1 tsp tandoori spice mix
   1/3 tsp fresh ginger, grated
   1/2 cup plain, non-fat yogurt

Mix yogurt, tandoori spice, cumin and ginger in a bowl. Brush mixture on chicken breasts. Grill on high for 2 minutes on each side. Reduce heat and cook 5 minutes longer on each side, basting while cooking.

Serve with 6 oz (3/4 cup) of cooked brown or wild rice and 1 cup of any of the following steamed vegetables: asparagus, broccoli, eggplant, green beans, kale, snow pea pods, or spinach.

1200 CALORIES

Week 2 * Day 6

BREAKFAST: One cup of cereal (see cereal choices) and one cup soy milk or low-fator skim milk.

MID-MORNING SNACK: Snacks may consist of one of the following choices: banana; apple; pear; 2 cups strawberries (no sugar added); 1.5 cups blueberries (no sugar added); 2 cups raspberries (no sugar added); low-calorie yogurt (100 calories); 1 oz of soy nuts (100 calories total, varies based on brand and preparation); 1 oz soy chips (I recommend Revival brand soy chips. Three to four times a week, if desired, you may substitute any 100-calorie food you desire, for example a part-skim mozzarella cheese stick or 1 oz of chocolate (100 calories).

LUNCH: Chicken Taquito
   8" whole-wheat tortilla wrap
   1 oz low-fat Cheddar cheese
   4 oz white chicken meat
   2 tsp salsa

   Heat in microwave or in toaster oven.

MID-AFTERNOON SNACK: Same as mid-morning snack.

DINNER: Shrimp Scampi, with rice and vegetable.

Family size (serves 4)	Single serving
4 tbsp butter (unsalted)	1 tbsp butter (unsalted)
4 tbsp olive oil	1 tbsp olive oil
6 large cloves garlic, minced	1-2 large cloves garlic, minced
1/2 cup chopped, fresh flat-leaf parsley	2 oz or 1/8 cup chopped, fresh flat-leaf parsley
juice of 1 lemon	juice of 1/4 lemon
1 cup dry white wine	2 oz or 1/4 cup dry white wine
2 pinches dried, hot red pepper flakes	1 pinch of dried, hot red pepper flakes
salt and black pepper to taste	salt and black pepper to taste
2 lbs large shrimp, shelled and de-veined, frozen or fresh	8 oz large shrimp, shelled and de-veined, frozen or fresh

Heat the butter and oil in a skillet over medium heat until the foam subsides. Add the garlic, parsley, lemon juice, wine, pepper flakes, salt and pepper. Bring to a boil, lower the heat, and simmer for 3 minutes. Add the shrimp to the skillet and cook, stirring frequently, for 5 to 6 minutes until the shrimp are pink. Remove from heat. Place the shrimp on a serving plate and pour the sauce from the skillet over them.

Serve immediately with 6 oz (3/4cup) of cooked brown or wild rice and 1 cup of any of the following steamed vegetables: asparagus, broccoli, eggplant, green beans, kale, snow peapods, or spinach.

1200 CALORIES

Week 2 * Day 7

BREAKFAST: One cup of cereal (see cereal choices) and one cup soy milk or low-fat or skim milk.

MID-MORNING SNACK: Snacks may consist of one of the following choices: banana; apple; pear; 2 cups strawberries (no sugar added); 1.5 cups blueberries (no sugar added); 2 cups raspberries (no sugar added); low-calorie yogurt (100 calories); 1 oz of soy nuts (100 calories total, varies based on brand and preparation); 1 oz soy chips (I recommend Revival brand soy chips. Three to four times a week, if desired, you may substitute any 100-calorie food you desire, for example a part-skim mozzarella cheese stick or 1 oz of chocolate (100 calories).

MID-MORNING SNACK: Same as mid-morning snack.

LUNCH: Vegetarian Greek Wrap
   8" whole-wheat tortilla wrap
   2 tbsp guacamole
   3 slices tomato
   2 oz hummus
   1 oz black olives
   2 oz cucumber
   1 oz feta cheese (reduced-fat)

MID-AFTERNOON SNACK: Same as mid-morning snack.

DINNER: Grilled Spicy Chicken Breast Fillets, with rice and vegetable.

Family size (Serves 4)	Single serving
1 small clove garlic, crushed	1 small clove garlic, crushed
1 small onion, finely chopped	1 small onion, finely chopped
2-3 tbsp lime juice	2-3 tbsp lime juice
2 tbsp olive oil	2 tbsp olive oil
1/2 tsp chili powder	1/2 tsp chili powder
fresh ground pepper to taste	fresh ground pepper to taste
4 - 6 oz boneless, skinless chicken breasts	1 - 6 oz boneless, skinless chicken breast

In a small bowl, combine ingredients. Coat chicken pieces thoroughly. On preheated grill or in broiler, cook chicken, turning once, 6-7 minutes, or until done.

Serve with 6 oz (3/4 cup) of cooked brown or wild rice and 1 cup of any of the following steamed vegetables: asparagus, broccoli, eggplant, green beans, kale, snow pea pods, or spinach.

1200 CALORIES

Week 3 * Day 1

BREAKFAST: One cup of cereal (see cereal choices) and one cup soy milk or low-fat or skim milk.

MID-MORNING SNACK: Snacks may consist of one of the following choices: banana; apple; pear; 2 cups strawberries (no sugar added); 1.5 cups blueberries (no sugar added); 2 cups raspberries (no sugar added); low-calorie yogurt (100 calories); 1 oz of soy nuts (100 calories total, varies based on brand and preparation); 1 oz soy chips (I recommend Revival brand soy chips. Three to four times a week, if desired, you may substitute any 100-calorie food you desire, for example a part-skim mozzarella cheese stick or 1 oz of chocolate (100 calories).

LUNCH: Ham and Cheese Wrap
   8" whole-wheat tortilla wrap
   4 oz Healthy Choice ham (low-fat ham)
   2 tsp mustard
   1 oz Cheddar cheese (low-fat if available)

MID-AFTERNOON SNACK: Same as mid-morning snack.

DINNER: Caribbean Grilled Tuna, with rice and vegetable.

Family size (serves 4)	Single serving
cooking oil spray	cooking oil spray
4 – 6 oz tuna steaks	1 - 6 oz tuna steak
1 tbsp lime and lemon juice	1 tsp lime and lemon juice
3 tbsp olive oil	1 tbsp olive oil
1 T of Caribbean Jerk Seasoning or Old Bay crab spice mixture	1 tsp Caribbean Jerk Seasoning or Old Bay crab spice mixture

Mix together juice, oil, and seasonings. Brush mixture onto tuna steaks. Spray pan with olive oil cooking spray. Preheat grill or broiler pan. Place tuna on broiler. Grill or broil 5 minutes per side or until fish flakes with a fork.

Serve with 1 cup of cooked brown or wild rice and 1 cup of any of the following steamed vegetables: asparagus, broccoli, eggplant, green beans, kale, snow pea pods, or spinach.

1200 CALORIES

Week 3 * Day 2

BREAKFAST: One cup of cereal (see cereal choices) and one cup soy milk or low-fat or skim milk.

MID-MORNING SNACK: Snacks may consist of one of the following choices: banana; apple; pear; 2 cups strawberries (no sugar added); 1.5 cups blueberries (no sugar added); 2 cups raspberries (no sugar added); low-calorie yogurt (100 calories); 1 oz of soy nuts (100 calories total, varies based on brand and preparation); 1 oz soy chips (I recommend Revival brand soy chips. Three to four times a week, if desired, you may substitute any 100-calorie food you desire, for example a part-skim mozzarella cheese stick or 1 oz of chocolate (100 calories).

LUNCH: Bar-B-Q Chicken Quesadilla
   8" whole-wheat tortilla wrap
   3 oz chicken
   2 tsp BBQ sauce
   1 1/2 oz reduced-fat cheddar cheese

MID-AFTERNOON SNACK: Same as mid-morning snack.

DINNER: Lemon Pepper Beef Steak, with baked potato and vegetable.

Family size (serves 4)	Single serving
1 1/2 lbs of lean beef sirloin tip round	5 oz lean beef sirloin tip round
1 tsp olive oil	1 tsp olive oil
2 garlic cloves, crushed	1 garlic clove, crushed
2 tsp oregano	1 tsp oregano
1/2 tsp lemon pepper salt	1/4 tsp lemon pepper salt

Combine seasoning ingredients in a bowl. Brush seasonings on steak. Broil steak until desired doneness.

Serve with 1 small (6 oz) baked potato, with 1 tsp soft canola margarine, and 1 cup of any of the following steamed vegetables: asparagus, broccoli, eggplant, green beans, kale, snow pea pods, or spinach.

1200 CALORIES

Week 3 * Day 3

BREAKFAST: One cup of cereal (see cereal choices) and one cup soy milk or low-fat or skim milk.

MID-MORNING SNACK: Snacks may consist of one of the following choices: banana; apple; pear; 2 cups strawberries (no sugar added); 1.5 cups blueberries (no sugar added); 2 cups raspberries (no sugar added); low-calorie yogurt (100 calories); 1 oz of soy nuts (100 calories total, varies based on brand and preparation); 1 oz soy chips (I recommend Revival brand soy chips. Three to four times a week, if desired, you may substitute any 100-calorie food you desire, for example a part-skim mozzarella cheese stick or 1 oz of chocolate (100 calories).

LUNCH: Garlic Chicken Burrito
   8" whole-wheat tortilla wrap
   2 oz chicken
   1 tsp garlic powder
   1 oz corn
   3 oz black beans
   3 lettuce leaves
   1 slice tomato
   1 tsp sour cream
   1 oz low-fat Mozzarella cheese

MID-AFTERNOON SNACK: Same as mid-morning snack.

DINNER: 2 Crab Cakes, with vegetable.

Family size (serves 4)
   1 egg beaten
   2 slices bread, crust removed, broken into crumbs
   1 tbsp seafood seasoning or Old Bay seasoning
   1 tsp Worcestershire sauce
   1 tbsp light mayonnaise
   1/2 tsp baking powder
   1 lb fresh crabmeat

Combine egg, breadcrumbs, seafood seasoning, Worcestershire sauce, mayonnaise and baking powder in a large bowl. Stir in crabmeat. Mix well. Shape mixture into 8 one-half inch thick patties. Broil for 10 minutes without turning.

Eat two crab cakes for a single serving (refrigerate or freeze the rest for later consumption) and serve with 1 cup of any of the following steamed vegetables: asparagus, broccoli, eggplant, green beans, kale, snow pea pods, or spinach.

1200 CALORIES

Week 3 * Day 4

BREAKFAST: One cup of cereal (see cereal choices) and one cup soy milk or low-fat or skim milk.

MID-MORNING SNACK: Snacks may consist of one of the following choices: banana; apple; pear; 2 cups strawberries (no sugar added); 1.5 cups blueberries (no sugar added); 2 cups raspberries (no sugar added); low-calorie yogurt (100 calories); 1 oz of soy nuts (100 calories total, varies based on brand and preparation); 1 oz soy chips (I recommend Revival brand soy chips. Three to four times a week, if desired, you may substitute any 100 calorie food you desire, for example a part-skim mozzarella cheese stick or 1 oz of chocolate (100 calories).

LUNCH: Shrimp and Avocado Wrap
   8" whole-wheat tortilla wrap
   4 oz shrimp fresh or frozen
   1/2 cup avocado, mashed

MID-AFTERNOON SNACK: Same as mid-morning snack.

DINNER: Gingered Beef and Broccoli, with rice.

Family size (serves 4)
   2 cups broccoli (keep stems 1/4 inch)
   1 cup cut snow peas
   1 red pepper, cut in half-inch pieces
   1/2 cup shitake mushrooms
   3/4 lb lean beef, cut for stir-fry
   3 tbsp water
   1.5 tbsp cornstarch
   2 tbsp olive oil
   1 tbsp fresh ginger, minced
   3/4 cup low-sodium soy sauce

Single serving
   1/4 of the above recipe (save the rest in refrigerator)

Add to a bowl the water, cornstarch, and soy sauce. Microwave broccoli, covered, on high power for 3 minutes. Heat non-stick skillet on high. When hot, pour 1 tsp olive oil into pan. Add ginger and beef and stir-fry until beef browns. Add sauce and toss to coat. Remove beef from pan. Add remaining oil. Add broccoli to pan along with peppers, mushrooms and snow peas. Stir-fry for 2 minutes. Return beef with sauce to pan, toss to evenly distribute.

Serve with 4 oz (1/2 cup) of brown rice.

1200 CALORIES

Week 3 * Day 5

BREAKFAST: One cup of cereal (see cereal choices) and one cup soy milk or low-fat or skim milk.

MID-MORNING SNACK: Snacks may consist of one of the following choices: banana; apple; pear; 2 cups strawberries (no sugar added); 1.5 cups blueberries (no sugar added); 2 cups raspberries (no sugar added); low-calorie yogurt (100 calories); 1 oz of soy nuts (100 calories total, varies based on brand and preparation); 1 oz soy chips (I recommend Revival brand soy chips. Three to four times a week, if desired, you may substitute any 100-calorie food you desire, for example a part-skim mozzarella cheese stick or 1 oz of chocolate (100 calories).

LUNCH: BBQ Pork Wrap
   8" whole-wheat tortilla wrap
   1 tsp onion powder
   2 tsp BBQ sauce
   2 tomato slices
   4 lettuce leaves
   4 oz pork loin

MID-AFTERNOON SNACK: Same as mid-morning snack.

DINNER: Lemon Baked Chicken, with rice and vegetable.

Family size (serves 4)	Single serving
Olive oil cooking spray	Olive oil cooking spray
2 tbsp fresh lemon juice	2 tsp fresh lemon juice
2 tbsp canola oil	2 tsp canola oil
1 clove of garlic, crushed	1/4 clove of garlic, crushed
1/2 tsp fresh ground pepper	fresh ground pepper to taste
2-2 1/2 lbs boneless, skinless chicken breasts	6 oz boneless, skinless chicken breast

Preheat oven to 350 degrees. Lightly spray a baking pan or a shallow casserole dish with cooking spray. In a small bowl, combine lemon juice, oil, garlic and pepper. Set aside. Rinse chicken and pat dry. Arrange chicken in prepared pan or dish. Pour lemon mixture over chicken pieces. Cover and bake for 40 minutes, or until tender, basting occasionally. Uncover and bake 10 minutes longer to allow chicken to brown.

Serve with 6 oz (3/4 cup) of cooked brown or wild rice and 1 cup of any of the following steamed vegetables asparagus, broccoli, eggplant, green beans, kale, snow pea pods, or spinach.

1200 CALORIES

Week 3 * Day 6

BREAKFAST: One cup of cereal (see cereal choices) and one cup soy milk or low-fat or skim milk.

MID-MORNING SNACK: Snacks may consist of one of the following choices: banana; apple; pear; 2 cups strawberries (no sugar added); 1.5 cups blueberries (no sugar added); 2 cups raspberries (no sugar added); low-calorie yogurt (100 calories); 1 oz of soy nuts (100 calories total, varies based on brand and preparation); 1 oz soy chips (I recommend Revival brand soy chips. Three to four times a week, if desired, you may substitute any 100-calorie food you desire, for example a part-skim mozzarella cheese stick or 1 oz of chocolate (100 calories).

LUNCH: Island Wrap
   8" whole-wheat tortilla wrap
   4 oz ham
   1 tsp bacon bits
   1 oz pineapple
   2 lettuce leaves
   3 slices tomato
   1 oz mozzarella cheese
   2 tsp fat-free ranch dressing

   MID-AFTERNOON SNACK: Same as mid-morning snack.

DINNER: Spinach Stuffed Sirloin

Family size (serves 4)	Single serving
1 1/2 lb lean sirloin steak, 1" to 1 1/2" thick	6 oz lean sirloin steak, 1" to 1 1/2" thick
1- 10 oz pkg frozen spinach, thawed and draine d	4 oz pkg frozen spinach, thawed and drained
2 cloves garlic, crushed	1/2 clove garlic, crushed
cooking oil spray	cooking oil spray
1/4 lb mushrooms, finely chopped	2 oz mushrooms, finely chopped
1/2 cup diced red bell pepper (optional)	2 oz diced red bell pepper (optional)
1 tbsp olive oil	1 tsp olive oil
1/4 cup grated Parmesan cheese	1 oz grated Parmesan cheese

Preheat broiler. Meanwhile, heat oil in small sauté pan until hot but not smoking. Cook garlic, mushroom, and red bell pepper until softened. Add spinach and heat through. Stir in grated Parmesan thoroughly and remove from heat. With a sharp knife, cut pocket in sirloin steak nearly to the edges. Stuff with warm spinach mixture and place on rack in shallow pan. For medium rare, broil for 5 minutes on first side and 3 minutes, approximately, after turning steak over. For other doneness, adjust broiling time accordingly.

Serve with 6 oz (3/4 cup) of cooked brown or wild rice and 1 cup of any of the following steamed vegetables asparagus, broccoli, eggplant, green beans, kale, snow pea pods, or spinach.

1200 CALORIES

Week 3 * Day 7

BREAKFAST: One cup of cereal (see cereal choices) and one cup soy milk or low fat or skim milk.

MID-MORNING SNACK: Snacks may consist of one of the following choices: banana; apple; pear; 2 cups strawberries (no sugar added); 1.5 cups blueberries (no sugar added); 2 cups raspberries (no sugar added); low-calorie yogurt (100 calories); 1 oz of soy nuts (100 calories total, varies based on brand and preparation); 1 oz soy chips (I recommend Revival brand soy chips. Three to four times a week, if desired, you may substitute any 100-calorie food you desire, for example a part-skim mozzarella cheese stick or 1 oz of chocolate (100 calories).

LUNCH: BBQ Pork Burrito

8" whole-wheat tortilla wrap	3 lettuce leaves
2 oz chicken	3 tomato slices
1 oz corn	1 oz low-fat mozzarella cheese
3 oz black beans	1 tsp barbeque sauce
1 tsp sour cream	

MID-AFTERNOON SNACK: Same as mid-morning snack.

DINNER: Chicken Manicotti, with rice and vegetable.

Family size (serves 4)	Single serving
3/4 tsp oregano	1/4 tsp oregano
1/2 tsp marjoram	1 pinch of marojram
3/4 tsp sweet basil	1/4 tsp sweet basil
1/4 tsp fresh ground pepper	1 pinch of fresh ground pepper
1- 6 oz can no-salt-added tomato paste	2 oz can no-salt-added tomato paste
1 cup water	2 oz water
1 clove garlic, minced	1/4 clove garlic, minced
4 boneless, skinless chicken breasts, (about 1 lb), fat removed	1 boneless, skinless chicken breast, (6 oz), fat removed
4 oz low-fat cottage cheese, drained	1 oz low-fat cottage cheese, drained
2 oz grated, part-skim mozzarella cheese	1 oz grated, part-skim mozzarella cheese

Preheat oven 350 degrees. In a small bowl, combine the four spices. Mix well. Set aside. In a small saucepan, blend tomato paste, water, and garlic. Add 3/4 of the seasoning mixture to the pan. Bring to a boil. Reduce heat and simmer 10 minutes, stirring occasionally. Meanwhile, rinse chicken and pat dry. Place fillets in a plastic bag and pound to 1/4" thickness. Set aside in a small bowl, combine remaining spice mixture with cottage cheese. Spoon mixtures onto centers of chicken breasts, leaving a 1/2 inch edge all around. From narrow end, roll each breast, leaving a1/2 inch edge all around. Spoon half of the tomato mixture into the bottom of a 10 x 6 inch baking dish. Arrange chicken roll on top, seam side down. Spoon remaining tomato mixture over the chicken rolls. Top with Mozzarella cheese and bake about 45 minutes, or until golden brown.

Serve with 6 oz (3/4 cup) of cooked brown or wild rice and 1 cup of any of the following steamed vegetables: asparagus, broccoli, eggplant, green beans, kale, snow pea pods, or spinach.

1400 CALORIE DIET

Calorie Distribution in 1400 Calorie Diet

Breakfast	250 Calories
Mid-Morning Snack	200 Calories
Lunch	375 Calories
Mid-Afternoon Snack	200 Calories
Dinner	375 Calories

Rules for the North Star Diet

1) Eat breakfast within 20 minutes after waking in the morning. Failure to eat a timely breakfast will decrease your fat-burning capacity, or metabolism. Breakfast choices consist of any high-fiber cereal with non-fat milk fortified with vitamin D and calcium or, preferably, non-fat soy milk fortified with vitamin D and calcium. High-fiber cereals should contain at least 8 grams of fiber in each serving. Recommended high-fiber cereals:

CEREAL	PORTION	CALORIES	FIBER (content)
General Mills Fiber One	1/2 cup	59	14 g
General Mills Fiber One Honey Clusters**	1 1/4 cup	170	14 g
Kellogg's Bran Buds	1/3 cup	80	11 g
Kellogg's All-Bran	1/2 cup	80	10 g
Post or Nabisco			
100% Bran	1/3 cup	80	9 g
Post Raisin Bran	1 cup	190	8 g
Kashi Good Friends	3/4 cup	90	8 g
Kashi Lean Crunch	1 cup	190	8 g
OATMEAL			
Quaker Weight Control	1 serving	160	8 g
TORTILLAS			
Cruz whole-wheat	large 8"	130	11 g
La tortilla factory	large 8"	80	14 g
Mission low carb	6" size	110	11 g

2) Consume mid-morning snacks and mid-afternoon snacks. Both snacks may consist of one (1200 calorie diet) or two (all other diets) of the following choices: banana; apple; pear; 2 cups strawberries (no sugar added); 1.5 cups blueberries (no sugar added); 2 cups raspberries (no sugar added); low-calorie yogurt (100 calories); 1 oz of soy nuts (100 calories total, varies based on brand and preparation); 1 oz soy chips (I recommend Revival brand soy chips). Failure to eat timely mid-morning and mid-afternoon snacks will decrease your fat-burning capacity, or metabloism. Three to four times a week you may substitute any food you desire(100 to 200 calories depending upon meal plan), for example one or two part-skim mozzarella cheese stick(s) or 1-2 oz of chocolate (100-200 calories).

Rules for the North Star Diet, cont'd.

3) Consume 2 liters of fluid a day (approximately 80 ounces). Eighty ounces of fluid is the equivalent of 8 ounces of water per hour for ten hours a day, or two 8-ounce glasses of water with each meal and snack. You may substitute diet soda pop or tea with meals if desired but no fruit juice or regular pop is allowed.

4) Consumption of two cups of green tea, one tea bag per cup, will promote 70 calories of weight loss on a daily basis. A personal favorite is Tazo Zen brand of green tea.

5) Consume dinner 3-4 hours prior to bedtime. If you eat closer to bedtime there is an increased chance the food will be stored and converted into fat while you sleep. If you are still hungry after dinner, you may consume an apple, pear or banana or 1 ounce of lean, grilled protein, e.g. turkey, ham, beef, or fish.

6) The meal plans are to be used as guides. Most individuals only eat 7-10 different foods in a given week. If yo u like certain wraps or dinners and not others, consume those you enjoy the most. I only ask that starting in the second week of the North Star Diet you begin utilizing a whole-wheat wrap/tortilla. (See lunch alternative if you desire to use bread as an alternative). Whole-wheat wraps can often contain as much as 10 –14 g of fiber per serving. They are easy to make. Combine fillings in the center of the tortilla and roll up. I recommend the following whole-wheat tortilla/wraps: Cruz brand whole-wheat tortilla (10 grams of dietary fiber per serving); La Tortilla Factory whol e-wheat, low-carb/low-fat tortillas (large size, 14 grams of fiber); and Carb Down flat bread (14 grams of fiber).

7) Consume daily: a multi-vitamin; 1200 mg of calcium carbonate; 1000 I.U. vitamin D; and 1000-3000 mg of fish oil.

** Personal Favorite

Measurement Conversions

Do not fear the measurements in the following calorie-specific diets. You could weigh each item as described. However, I approximate all food quantities based on the volume of a deck of playing cards.

3 ounces (oz) = the fluid volume of a deck of playing cards.

1 cup = 8 fluid ounces = 2.5 fluid equivalents of a deck of playing cards.

1 ounce (oz) = the fluid equivalent of one-third of a deck of playing cards.

1/2 ounce (oz) = 1 tablespoon (tbsp) = the fluid equivalent of 1/6 of a deck of playing cards.

1400 CALORIES

Week 1 * Day 1

BREAKFAST: One cup of cereal (see cereal choices) and one cup soy milk or low-fat or skim milk.

MID-MORNING SNACK: Snacks may consist of two of the following choices: banana; apple; pear; 2 cups strawberries (no sugar added); 1.5 cups blueberries (no sugar added); 2 cups raspberries (no sugar added); low-calorie yogurt (100 calories); 1 oz of soy nuts (100 calories total, varies based on brand and preparation); 1 oz soy chips (I recommend Revival brand soy chips. Three to four times a week, if desired, you may substitute any 200-calorie food you desire, for example two part-skim mozzarella cheese sticks or 2 oz of chocolate (200 calories).

LUNCH: Mediterranean Wrap
   8" tortilla wrap
   4 oz turkey, roasted or sliced, skinless white meat
   4 lettuce leaves
   2 oz cucumber strips
   1 tsp red pepper flakes
   1 oz feta cheese
   2 tsp fat-free red wine vinegar

MID-AFTERNOON SNACK: Same as mid-morning snack.

DINNER: Crispy Baked Chicken, with rice and vegetable.

Family size (4 servings)	Single serving
2-2.5 lbs boneless, skinless chicken breasts	6 oz boneless, skinless chicken breast
1 cup skim milk	1/4 cup skim milk
1 cup cornflake crumbs	1/4 cup cornflake crumbs
1 tsp rosemary	1 pinch rosemary
1 tsp fresh ground black pepper	1 pinch fresh ground black pepper
Pam cooking oil spray	Pam cooking oil spray or olive oil spray

Preheat oven to 350 degrees. Cover a baking dish with foil and spray lightly with cooking oil spray. Rinse chicken and pat dry. Set aside. Pour milk into a shallow bowl. Combine cornflake crumbs, rosemary, and pepper in another shallow bowl. Dip chicken first into milk and then into crumb mixture. Allow to stand briefly so coating will adhere. Arrange chicken in prepared pan so pieces do not touch. Bake 40 minutes or until done. Crumbs will form a crisp "skin".

Serve with 3/4 cup of cooked wild or brown rice and 1 cup of any of the following steamed vegetables: asparagus, broccoli, eggplant, green beans, kale, snow pea pods, or spinach.

1400 CALORIES

Week 1 * Day 2

BREAKFAST: One cup of cereal (see cereal choices) and one cup soy milk or low-fat or skim milk.

MID-MORNING SNACK: Snacks may consist of two of the following choices: banana; apple; pear; 2 cups strawberries (no sugar added); 1.5 cups blueberries (no sugar added); 2 cups raspberries (no sugar added); low-calorie yogurt (100 calories); 1 oz of soy nuts (100 calories total, varies based on brand and preparation); 1 oz soy chips (I recommend Revival brand soy chips. Three to four times a week, if desired, you may substitute any 200-calorie food you desire, for example two part-skim mozzarella cheese sticks or 2 oz of chocolate (200 calories).

LUNCH: Beef Taquito Wrap
  8" tortilla wrap
  4 oz round steak, trimmed
  1 oz mozzarella low-fat cheese
  2 tsp salsa

MID-AFTERNOON SNACK: Same as mid-morning snack.

DINNER: Scallops Oriental, with rice and vegetable.

Family size (4 servings)	Single serving
cooking oil spray (preferably olive oil)	cooking oil spray (preferably olive oil)
1 lb fresh or frozen scallops	4 oz of fresh or frozen scallops
1/8 cup honey	2 tsp honey
1/8 cup mustard	2 tsp mustard
1/2 tsp curry powder	pinch of curry powder
1/2 tsp lemon juice	1/8 tsp lemon juice

Preheat broiler. Lightly spray baking pan with cooking spray. Rinse scallops and drain. Place in a baking pan. In a saucepan, combine remaining ingredients. Brush scallops with sauce. Broil 4 inches from heat for 5-8 minutes or until browned.

Serve with 3/4 cup of cooked wild or brown rice and 1 cup of any of the following steamed vegetables: asparagus, broccoli, eggplant, green beans, kale, snow pea pods, or spinach.

1400 CALORIES

Week 1 * Day 3

BREAKFAST: One cup of cereal (see cereal choices) and one cup soy milk or low-fat or skim milk.

MID-MORNING SNACK: Snacks may consist of two of the following choices: banana; apple; pear; 2 cups strawberries (no sugar added); 1.5 cups blueberries (no sugar added); 2 cups raspberries (no sugar added); low-calorie yogurt (100 calories); 1 oz of soy nuts (100 calories total, varies based on brand and preparation); 1 oz soy chips (I recommend Revival brand soy chips. Three to four times a week, if desired, you may substitute any 200-calorie food you desire, for example two part-skim mozzarella cheese sticks or 2 oz of chocolate (200 calories).

LUNCH: Tuna Mayo Wrap
   8" tortilla wrap
   1.5 oz low fat mayonnaise
   6 0z tuna
   1/4 stick celery

MID-AFTERNOON SNACK: Same as mid-morning snack.

DINNER: Tomato, Mushroom, and Jack Cheese Omelet, with vegetable and baked potato.

Single Serving
   Cooking oil spray (olive oil preferable)
   2 eggs or egg substitute equivalent
   1/4 cup seeded, chopped tomato
   1/2 oz shredded, low-fat Monterey Jack cheese
   1/4 cup mushrooms
   1 tsp chopped cilantro or parsley
   Hot pepper sauce (optional)

Spray skillet with cooking oil, or use non-stick frying pan. Place pan over medium-high heat. In a small bowl, place eggs or egg substitute . Beat and pour mixture into pan. Stir eggs in a circular motion. Do not scrape bottom of pan. When the omelet is almost cooked, add fillings. Fold omelet over with a fork while holding the pan at 45-degree angle. Roll omelet onto plate and serve.

Serve with 1 medium (7 oz) baked potato, with 1 tsp soft canola margarine, and 1 cup of any of the following steamed vegetables: asparagus, broccoli, eggplant, green beans, kale, snow pea pods, or spinach.

1400 CALORIES

Week 1 * Day 4

BREAKFAST: One cup of cereal (see cereal choices) and one cup soy milk or low-fat or skim milk.

MID-MORNING SNACK: Snacks may consist of two of the following choices: banana; apple; pear; 2 cups strawberries (no sugar added); 1.5 cups blueberries (no sugar added); 2 cups raspberries (no sugar added); low-calorie yogurt (100 calories); 1 oz of soy nuts (100 calories total, varies based on brand and preparation); 1 oz soy chips (I recommend Revival brand soy chips. Three to four times a week, if desired, you may substitute any 200-calorie food you desire, for example two part-skim mozzarella cheese sticks or 2 oz of chocolate (200 calories).

LUNCH: Beef Wrap
   8" tortilla wrap
   4 oz broiled, trimmed round steak
   1/2 cup of raw or broiled mushrooms
   2 tsp Worcestershire sauce
   1 tsp soy sauce

MID-AFTERNOON SNACK: Same as mid-morning snack.

DINNER: Mustard-Crusted Pork, with rice and vegetable.

Serving for two
   2 tsp soy or tofu flour (available at most health food stores)
   1 tsp mustard powder
   1/2 tsp pepper
   1/4 cup olive oil
   1 lb boneless, center-cut pork chops, cut against the grain into 3" strips, about 3/8 " thick

Single serving
   2 tsp soy or tofu flour (available at most health food stores)
   1 tsp mustard powder
   1/2 tsp pepper
   1/4 cup olive oil
   8 oz boneless, center-cut pork chops, cut against the grain into 3" strips, about 3/8 " thick

Combine the flour, mustard powder, and pepper in a bowl and mix well. Dust the pork with the flour mixture. Heat 2 tbs oil over medium heat until hot but not smoking. Add half the pork and brown for five minutes on each side, or until cooked through. Repeat with the remaining pork. Sprinkle with seasoning. Remove from he at and serve immediately.

Serve with 3/4 cup of cooked wild or brown rice and 1 cup of any of the following steamed vegetables: asparagus, broccoli, eggplant, green beans, kale, snow pea pods, or spinach.

1400 CALORIES

Week 1 * Day 5

BREAKFAST: One cup of cereal (see cereal choices) and one cup soy milk or low-fat or skim milk.

MID-MORNING SNACK: Snacks may consist of two of the following choices: banana; apple; pear; 2 cups strawberries (no sugar added); 1.5 cups blueberries (no sugar added); 2 cups raspberries (no sugar added); low-calorie yogurt (100 calories); 1 oz of soy nuts (100 calories total, varies based on brand and preparation); 1 oz soy chips (I recommend Revival brand soy chips. Three to four times a week, if desired, you may substitute any 200-calorie food you desire, for example two part-skim mozzarella cheese sticks or 2 oz of chocolate (200 calories).

LUNCH: Turkey Vegetable Wrap
   8" tortilla wrap
   4 oz turkey, roasted or sliced, skin less white meat
   1 oz corn, canned in water
   1 oz red pepper
   1 oz green onion
   2 tsp fat-free, light ranch dressing

MID-AFTERNOON SNACK: Same as mid-morning snack.

DINNER: Fish Fillets with Asparagus, with rice and vegetable.

Family size (serves four)	Single serving
Cooking oil spray (preferably olive oil)	Cooking oil spray (preferably olive oil)
4 - 5 oz mild, white fish fillets (Haddock, cod, etc.)	1 - 5 oz mild, white fish fillet (Haddock, cod, etc.)
1/2 tsp ground black pepper	1/4 tsp ground black pepper
2 tbsp unsalted butter	1 tbsp unsalted butter
12 stalks cooked asparagus	3 stalks cooked asparagus
1/3 cup tangy sour cream	1/3 cup tangy sour cream
1/3 cup plain low-fat yogurt	1/3 cup plain low-fat yogurt
2 tsp minced chives	1 tsp minced chives
2 tsp horseradish	1 tsp horseradish
1 egg white	1 egg white
2 tsp chopped parsley	1 tsp chopped parsley

Preheat broiler. Lightly spray broiler pan with cooking spray. Rinse fish and pat dry. Season fish with pepper and lemon juice and brush with margarine. Place on broiler pan and broil about 8 minutes or until fish almost flakes. Remove from oven and top each fillet with 3 stalks of asparagus. In a small bowl, combine sour cream, yogurt, chives, horseradish, and dill weed. In another bowl, beat egg whites until stiff peaks form; fold into sour cream mixture. Spread mixture over each fillet to cover fish and asparagus. Return to broiler and broil 1-2 minutes, or until golden brown. Sprinkle with parsley.

Serve with 3/4 cup of cooked wild or brown rice and 1 cup of any of the following steamed vegetables: asparagus, broccoli, eggplant, green beans, kale, snow pea pods, or spinach.

1400 CALORIES

Week 1 * Day 6

BREAKFAST: One cup of cereal (see cereal choices) and one cup soy milk or low-fat or skim milk.

MID-MORNING SNACK: Snacks may consist of two of the following choices: banana; apple; pear; 2 cups strawberries (no sugar added); 1.5 cups blueberries (no sugar added); 2 cups raspberries (no sugar added); low-calorie yogurt (100 calories); 1 oz of soy nuts (100 calories total, varies based on brand and preparation); 1 oz soy chips (I recommend Revival brand soy chips. Three to four times a week, if desired, you may substitute any 200-calorie food you desire, for example two part-skim mozzarella cheese sticks or 2 oz of chocolate (200 calories).

LUNCH: California Chicken Wrap
   8" tortilla wrap
   3 oz grilled white chicken
   2 tsp guacamole
   3 slices tomato
   3 leaves lettuce
   1 tsp bacon bits

MID-AFTERNOON SNACK: Same as mid-morning snack.

DINNER: Feta Burgers, with rice and steamed vegetable.

Family size (serves 4)
   cooking oil spray, preferably olive oil
   1 lb ground sirloin or ground round
   1/4 cup crumbled feta cheese
   1/4 cup finely chopped black olives
   1/2 tsp salt
   1/2 tsp. pepper

Single serving
   4 oz ground sirloin or ground round
   1 oz Feta cheese
   1 oz finely chopped black olives
   pinch of salt
   pepper to taste

Heat pan sprayed with cooking spray. Mix remaining ingredients and shape into four patties (one for single serving). Sauté patties at medium high heat for 5 minutes on each side or to desired doneness.

Serve with 3/4 cup of cooked wild or brown rice and 1 cup of any of the following steamed vegetables: asparagus, broccoli, eggplant, green beans, kale, snow peapods, or spinach.

1400 CALORIES

Week 1 * Day 7

BREAKFAST: One cup of cereal (see cereal choices) and one cup soy milk or low-fat or skim milk.

MID-MORNING SNACK: Snacks may consist of two of the following choices: banana; apple; pear; 2 cups strawberries (no sugar added); 1.5 cups blueberries (no sugar added); 2 cups raspberries (no sugar added); low-calorie yogurt (100 calories); 1 oz of soy nuts (100 calories total, varies based on brand and preparation); 1 oz soy chips (I recommend Revival brand soy chips. Three to four times a week, if desired, you may substitute any 200-calorie food you desire, for example two part-skim mozzarella cheese sticks or 2 oz of chocolate (200 calories).

LUNCH: Ham Club Wrap
   8" tortilla wrap
   4 oz ham
   3 tomato slices
   3 lettuce leaves
   1 tsp bacon bits
   1 tsp light Italian dressing
   1 oz low-fat mozzarella cheese

MID-AFTERNOON SNACK: Same as mid-morning snack.

DINNER: Lemon Baked Chicken, with rice and steamed vegetable.

Family size (serves 4)	Single serving
olive oil cooking spray	olive oil cooking spray
2 tsp fresh lemon juice	1 tsp fresh lemon juice
2 tsp low-fat margarine or safflower oil	1 tsp low-fat margarine or safflower oil
1 clove garlic, crushed	1/4 clove garlic, crushed
1/2 tsp fresh ground black pepper	1/8 tsp fresh ground black pepper
2–2.5 lbs of boneless, skinless chicken breast.	6 oz boneless, skinless chicken breast

Preheat oven to 350 degrees. Lightly spray a baking pan or a shallow casserole dish with cooking spray. In a small bowl, combine lemon juice, oil, garlic and pepper. Set aside. Rinse chicken and pat dry. Arrange chicken in prepared pan or dish. Pour lemon mixture over chicken pieces. Cover and bake 40 minutes or until tender, basting occasionally. Uncover and bake 10 minutes longer to allow chicken to brown.

Serve with 3/4 cup of cooked wild or brown rice and 1 cup of any of the following steamed vegetables: asparagus, broccoli, eggplant, green beans, kale, snow pea pods, or spinach.

1400 CALORIES

Week 2 * Day 1

BREAKFAST: One cup of cereal (see cereal choices) and one cup soy milk or low-fat or skim milk.

MID-MORNING SNACK: Snacks may consist of two of the following choices: banana; apple; pear; 2 cups strawberries (no sugar added); 1.5 cups blueberries (no sugar added); 2 cups raspberries (no sugar added); low-calorie yogurt (100 calories); 1 oz of soy nuts (100 calories total, varies based on brand and preparation); 1 oz soy chips (I recommend Revival brand soy chips. Three to four times a week, if desired, you may substitute any 200-calorie food you desire, for example two part-skim mozzarella cheese sticks or 2 oz of chocolate (200 calories).

LUNCH: Chicken with Zucchini and Roasted Pepper Wrap
   8" whole-wheat tortilla wrap
   4 oz broiled white chicken meat
   3-4 oz zucchini
   2 oz pickled sweet peppers
   1 oz part-skim, reduced-fat mozzarella cheese

MID-AFTERNOON SNACK: Same as mid-morning snack.

DINNER: Pineapple and Shrimp, with rice and vegetable

Family size (Serves 4)
   1 clove garlic
   2 tbsp canola margarine
   1/4 cup honey
   1 tbsp sweet chili sauce
   1 tbsp soy sauce
   1 whole pineapple, or 20 oz canned in water or light syrup
   2 lbs shrimp, fresh or frozen, peeled and de-veined

Single serving
   1 tsp garlic powder or 1/4 clove of garlic
   2 tsp canola margarine
   1 oz honey
   1 tsp sweet chili sauce
   1 tsp of soy sauce
   6 oz fresh pineapple, or 6 oz canned in water or light syrup
   6 oz shrimp, fresh or frozen, peeled and de-veined

Combine first five ingredients in a bowl. Brush shrimp with the mixture. Grill at high temperature for 5 minutes.

Serve with 3/4 cup of cooked wild or brown rice and 1 cup of any of the following steamed vegetables: asparagus, broccoli, eggplant, green beans, kale, snow pea pods, or spinach.

1400 CALORIES

Week 2 * Day 2

BREAKFAST: One cup of cereal (see cereal choices) and one cup soy milk or low-fat or skim milk.

MID-MORNING SNACK: Snacks may consist of two of the following choices: banana; apple; pear; 2 cups strawberries (no sugar added); 1.5 cups blueberries (no sugar added); 2 cups raspberries (no sugar added); low-calorie yogurt (100 calories); 1 oz of soy nuts (100 calories total, varies based on brand and preparation); 1 oz soy chips (I recommend Revival brand soy chips. Three to four times a week, if desired, you may substitute any 200-calorie food you desire, for example two part-skim mozzarella cheese sticks or 2 oz of chocolate (200 calories).

LUNCH: Santa Fe Steak Burrito
  8" whole-wheat tortilla wrap
  2 oz steak
  1 oz corn
  3 oz black beans
  1 tsp sour cream
  3 lettuce leaves
  3 tomato slices
  1 oz low-fat mozzarella cheese
  2 tsp salsa

MID-AFTERNOON SNACK: Same as mid-morning snack.

DINNER: Turkey Burgers, with wild rice and vegetable.

Family size (serves 4)	Single serving
1 lb ground turkey (90% lean), raw, thawed	4 oz ground turkey (90% lean), raw, thawed
1/4 cup onions, or powdered onion flakes	1 oz onions, or powdered onion flakes
2 tbsp green peppers	2 tsp green peppers
1 tbsp Worcestershire Sauce	1 tsp Worcestershire sauce
2 tbsp ketchup	1 tsp ketchup
1/4 tsp black pepper	1/8 tsp black pepper
lettuce leaves	lettuce leaves
tomato slices	tomato slices
4 whole-wheat pita pockets	1 whole-wheat pita pocket

Form ground turkey and seasoning into patties. Grill or broil for 5 minutes per side, or until done. Top patties with lettuce and tomato and place in pita pocket.

Serve with 4 oz (1/2 cup) of cooked brown or wild rice and 1 cup of any of the following steamed vegetables: asparagus, broccoli, eggplant, green beans, kale, snow pea pods, or spinach.

1400 CALORIES

Week 2 *Day 3

BREAKFAST: One cup of cereal (see cereal choices) and one cup soy milk or low-fat or skim milk.

MID-MORNING SNACK: Snacks may consist of two of the following choices: banana; apple; pear; 2 cups strawberries (no sugar added); 1.5 cups blueberries (no sugar added); 2 cups raspberries (no sugar added); low-calorie yogurt (100 calories); 1 oz of soy nuts (100 calories total, varies based on brand and preparation); 1 oz soy chips (I recommend Revival brand soy chips. Three to four times a week, if desired, you may substitute any 200-calorie food you desire, for example two part-skim mozzarella cheese sticks or 2 oz of chocolate (200 calories).

LUNCH: Tasty Turkey Wrap
   8" whole-wheat tortilla wrap
   onion powder to taste
   4 oz turkey
   2 tsp olives
   1 oz mozzarella low-fat cheese
   2 tsp fat-free mayo
   3 lettuce leaves
   1 tsp mustard
   3 slices tomato

MID-AFTERNOON SNACK: Same as mid-morning snack.

DINNER: Chicken with Mushrooms, with baked potato and vegetable.

Family size (serves 4)	Single serving
4 - 6 oz chicken breasts, skinless	6 oz chicken breast, skinless
20 oz button mushrooms	5 oz button mushrooms
1/2 tsp pepper	1/4 tsp pepper
2 cloves garlic, crushed	1 garlic clove, crushed
2 tbsp olive oil	1 tbsp olive oil
juice of half a lemon	juice of 1/4 lemon
1 cup dry white wine	1/4 cup dry white wine
pinch of dried hot red pepper flakes	pinch of dried hot red pepper flakes

Grill chicken, set aside. Heat oil in a heavy skillet over medium heat. Add the garlic, lemon juice, wine, pepper, and red pepper flakes. Bring to a boil. Lower heat and add mushrooms. Simmer and stir frequently for 5–6 minutes. Add pre-grilled chicken.

Serve with 1 medium (7 oz) baked potato with 1 tsp soft canola margarine, and 1 cup of any of the following steamed vegetables: asparagus, broccoli, eggplant, greenbeans, kale, snow pea pods, or spinach.

1400 CALORIES

Week 2 * Day 4

BREAKFAST: One cup of cereal (see cereal choices) and one cup soy milk or low-fat or skim milk.

MID-MORNING SNACK: Snacks may consist of two of the following choices: banana; apple; pear; 2 cups strawberries (no sugar added); 1.5 cups blueberries (no sugar added); 2 cups raspberries (no sugar added); low-calorie yogurt (100 calories); 1 oz of soy nuts (100 calories total, varies based on brand and preparation); 1 oz soy chips (I recommend Revival brand soy chips. Three to four times a week, if desired, you may substitute any 200-calorie food you desire, for example two part-skim mozzarella cheese sticks or 2 oz of chocolate (200 calories).

LUNCH: Greek Wrap
   8" whole-wheat tortilla wrap
   4 oz grilled chicken breast, no skin
   1 oz feta cheese (reduced-fat)
   4 lettuce leaves
   2-3 tomato slices
   2 tsp low-calorie vinaigrette dressing

MID-AFTERNOON SNACK: Same as mid-morning snack.

DINNER: Pork with Green Chile and Cheese, and rice and vegetable.

Family size (serves 4)
   1.5 lbs boneless, center-cut loin pork chops or sirloin pork steaks (fat removed)
   2 tbsp olive oil
   1/2 cup green chili salsa
   3/4 cup low-fat cheese, shredded (Feta, Muenster, Cheddar, or Mozzarella)

Single serving
   6 oz boneless, center cut loin pork chop s or sirloin pork steaks (fat removed)
   1 tsp olive oil
   2 oz green chili salsa
   2 oz low-fat cheese, shredded (feta, Muenster, cheddar, or mozzarella)

Heat oil in pan over medium heat until hot but not smoking. Add pork to pan and brown for 3-5 minutes. Turn heat to low, add 1/2 cup water, and cover pan. Cook for 20-25 minutes or until water is nearly evaporated. Pour salsa over pork, covering evenly. Sprinkle with shredded cheese, cover and cook for additional 3 to 5 minutes or until salsa is heated and cheese is melted.

Serve immediately with 6 oz (3/4 cup) of cooked brown or wild rice and 1 cup of any of the following steamed vegetables: asparagus, broccoli, eggplant, green beans, kale, snow pea pods, or spinach.

1400 CALORIES

Week 2 * Day 5

BREAKFAST: One cup of cereal (see cereal choices) and one cup soy milk or low-fat or skim milk.

MID-MORNING SNACK: Snacks may consist of two of the following choices: banana; apple; pear; 2 cups strawberries (no sugar added); 1.5 cups blueberries (no sugar added); 2 cups raspberries (no sugar added); low-calorie yogurt (100 calories); 1 oz of soy nuts (100 calories total, varies based on brand and preparation); 1 oz soy chips (I recommend Revival brand soy chips. Three to four times a week, if desired, you may substitute any 200-calorie food you desire, for example two part-skim mozzarella cheese sticks or 2 oz of chocolate (200 calories).

LUNCH: Bean and Cheese Burrito
   8" whole-wheat tortilla wrap
   2 oz reduced-fat cheddar cheese
   5 oz black beans
   3 lettuce leaves

Heat, if desired, in mi crowave or toaster oven.

MID-AFTERNOON SNACK: Same as mid-morning snack.

DINNER: Tandoori Chicken, with rice and vegetable.

Family Size (serves 4)
   4 - 6 oz chicken breasts, skinless
   3 tsp tandoori spice mix
   1 tsp fresh ginger, grated
   1 1/2 cups plain, non-fat yogurt

Single serving
   1 - 6 oz chicken breast, skinless
   1 tsp tandoori spice mix
   1/3 tsp fresh ginger, grated
   1/2 cup plain, non-fat yogurt

Mix yogurt, tandoori spice, cumin and ginger in a bowl. Brush mixture on chicken breasts. Grill on high for 2 minutes on each side. Reduce heat and cook 5 minutes longer on each side, basting while cooking.

Serve with 6 oz (3/4 cup) of cooked brown or wild rice and 1 cup of any of the following steamed vegetables: asparagus, broccoli, eggplant, gree n beans, kale, snow pea pods, or spinach.

1400 CALORIES

Week 2 * Day 6

BREAKFAST: One cup of cereal (see cereal choices) and one cup soy milk or low-fat or skim milk.

MID-MORNING SNACK: Snacks may consist of two of the following choices: banana; apple; pear; 2 cups strawberries (no sugar added); 1.5 cups blueberries (no sugar added); 2 cups raspberries (no sugar added); low-calorie yogurt (100 calories); 1 oz of soy nuts (100 calories total, varies based on brand and preparation); 1 oz soy chips (I recommend Revival brand soy chips. Three to four times a week, if desired, you may substitute any 200-calorie food you desire, for example two part-skim mozzarella cheese sticks or 2 oz of chocolate (200 calories).

LUNCH: Chicken Taquito
   8" whole-wheat tortilla wrap
   1 oz low-fat cheddar cheese
   4 oz white chicken meat
   2 tsp salsa

   Heat in microwave or in toaster oven

MID-AFTERNOON SNACK: Same as mid-morning snack.

DINNER: Shrimp Scampi, wi th rice and vegetable.

Family size (serves 4)	Single serving
4 tbsp butter (unsalted)	1tbsp butter (unsalted)
4 tbsp olive oil	1 tbsp olive oil
6 large cloves garlic, minced	1-2 large cloves garlic minced
1/2 cup chopped, fresh flat-leaf parsley	2 oz or 1/8 cup chopped fresh flat-leaf parsley
juice of 1 lemon	juice of 1/4 lemon
1 cup dry white wine	2 oz or 1/4 cup of dry white wine
2 pinches of dried, hot red pepper flakes	1 pinch of dried, hot red pepper flakes
salt and black pepper to taste	salt and black pepper to taste
2 lbs large shrimp, shelled and de-veined, frozen or fresh	8 oz large shrimp, shelled and de-veined, frozen or fresh

Heat the butter and oil in a skillet over medium heat until the foam subsides. Add the garlic, parsley, lemon juice, wine, pepper flakes, salt and pepper. Bring to a boil, lower the heat, and simmer for 3 minutes. Add the shrimp to the skillet and cook, stirring frequently, for 5 to 6 minutes until the shrimp are pink. Remove from heat. Place the shrimp on a serving plate and pour the sauce from the skillet over them. Serve immediately with 6 oz (3/4 cup) of cooked brown or wild rice and 1 cup of any of the following steamed vegetables: asparagus, broccoli, eggplant, greenbeans, kale, snow pea pods, or spinach.

Serve immediately with 6 oz (3/4cup) of cooked brown or wild rice and 1 cup of any of the following steamed vegetables: asparagus, broccoli, eggplant, greenbeans, kale, snow peapods, or spinach.

1400 CALORIES

Week 2 * Day 7

BREAKFAST: One cup of cereal (see cereal choices) and one cup soy milk or low-fat or skim milk.

MID-MORNING SNACK: Snacks may consist of two of the following choices: banana; apple; pear; 2 cups strawberries (no sugar added); 1.5 cups blueberries (no sugar added); 2 cups raspberries (no sugar added); low-calorie yogurt (100 calories); 1 oz of soy nuts (100 calories total, varies based on brand and preparation); 1 oz soy chips (I recommend Revival brand soy chips. Three to four times a week, if desired, you may substitute any 200-calorie food you desire, for example two part-skim mozzarella cheese sticks or 2 oz of chocolate (200 calories).

LUNCH: Vegetarian Greek Wrap
   8" whole-wheat tortilla wrap
   1 oz black olives
   2 tbsp guacamole
   2 oz cucumber
   3 tomato slices
   1 oz feta cheese (reduced-fat)
   2 oz hummus

MID-AFTERNOON SNACK: Same as mid-morning snack.

DINNER: Grilled Spicy Chicken Breast Fillets, with rice and vegetable.

Family size (Serves 4)	Single serving
1 small clove garlic, crushed	1/4 small clove garlic, crushed
1 small onion, finely chopped	1/4 small onion, finely chopped
2-3 tbsp lime juice	1 tbsp lime juice
2 tbsp olive oil	1 tbsp olive oil
1/2 tsp chili powder	pinch chili powder
fresh ground pepper to taste	fresh ground pepper to taste
4 - 6 oz boneless, skinless chicken breasts	1 - 6 oz boneless, skinless chicken breast

In a small bowl, combine ingredients. Coat chicken pieces thoroughly. On preheated grill or in broiler, cook chicken, turning once, 6-7 minutes, or until done.

Serve with 6 oz (3/4 cup) of cooked brown or wild rice and 1 cup of any of the following steamed vegetables: asparagus, broccoli, eggplant, green beans, kale, snow pea pods, or spinach.

1400 CALORIES

Week 3 * Day 1

BREAKFAST: One cup of cereal (see cereal choices) and one cup soy milk or low-fat or skim milk.

MID-MORNING SNACK: Snacks may consist of two of the following choices: banana; apple; pear; 2 cups strawberries (no sugar added); 1.5 cups blueberries (no sugar added); 2 cups raspberries (no sugar added); low-calorie yogurt (100 calories); 1 oz of soy nuts (100 calories total, varies based on brand and preparation); 1 oz soy chips (I recommend Revival brand soy chips. Three to four times a week, if desired, you may substitute any 200-calorie food you desire, for example two part-skim mozzarella cheese sticks or 2 oz of chocolate (200 calories).

LUNCH: Ham and Cheese Wrap
   8" whole-wheat tortilla wrap
   4 oz Healthy Choice ham (low-fat ham)
   2 tsp mustard
   1 oz cheddar cheese (low-fat if available)

MID-AFTERNOON SNACK: Same as mid-morning snack.

DINNER: Caribbean Grilled Tuna, with rice and vegetable.

Family size (serves 4)
   cooking oil spray
   4 – 6 oz tuna steaks
   1 tbsp lime and lemon juice
   3 tbsp olive oil
   1 tbsp Caribbean Jerk Seasoning or Old Bay crab spice mixture

Single serving
   cooking oil spray
   6 oz tuna steak
   1 tsp lime and lemon juice
   1 tbsp olive oil
   1 tsp Caribbean Jerk Seasoning or Old Bay crab spice mixture

Mix together juice, oil, and seasonings. Brush mixture onto tuna steaks. Spray pan with olive oil cooking spray. Preheat grill or broiler pan. Place tuna on broiler. Grill or broil 5 minutes per side or until fish flakes with a fork.

Serve with 1 cup of cooked brown or wild rice an d 1 cup of any of the following steamed vegetables: asparagus, broccoli, eggplant, green beans, kale, snow pea pods, or spinach.

1400 CALORIES

Week 3 * Day 2

BREAKFAST: One cup of cereal (see cereal choices) and one cup soy milk or low-fat or skim milk.

MID-MORNING SNACK: Snacks may consist of two of the following choices: banana; apple; pear; 2 cups strawberries (no sugar added); 1.5 cups blueberries (no sugar added); 2 cups raspberries (no sugar added); low-calorie yogurt (100 calories); 1 oz of soy nuts (100 calories total, varies based on brand and preparation); 1 oz soy chips (I recommend Revival brand soy chips. Three to four times a week, if desired, you may substitute any 200-calorie food you desire, for example two part-skim mozzarella cheese sticks or 2 oz of chocolate (200 calories).

LUNCH: Bar-B-Q Chicken Quesadilla
   8" whole-wheat tortilla wrap
   3 oz chicken
   2 tsp BBQ sauce
   1 1/2 oz reduced-fat cheddar cheese

MID-AFTERNOON SNACK: Same as mid-morning snack.

DINNER: Lemon Pepper Beef Steak, with baked potato and vegetable.

Family size (serves 4)
   1 1/2 lbs of lean beef steak, sirloin tip or round
   1 tsp olive oil
   2 garlic cloves, crushed
   2 tsp oregano
   1/2 tsp lemon pepper salt

Single serving
   5 oz lean beef steak, sirloin tip or round
   1 tsp olive oil
   1 garlic clove, crushed
   1 tsp oregano
   1/4 tsp lemon pepper salt

Combine seasoning ingredients in a bowl. Brush seasonings on steak. Broil steak until desired doneness.

Serve with 1 small (6 oz) baked potato, with 1 tsp soft canola margarine, and 1 cup of any of the following steamed vegetables: asparagus, broccoli, eggplant, green beans, kale, snow pea pods, or spinach.

1400 CALORIES

Week 3 * Day 3

BREAKFAST: One cup of cereal (see cereal choices) and one cup soy milk or low-fat or skim milk.

MID-MORNING SNACK: Snacks may consist of two of the following choices: banana; apple; pear; 2 cups strawberries (no sugar added); 1.5 cups blueberries (no sugar added); 2 cups raspberries (no sugar added); low-calorie yogurt (100 calories); 1 oz of soy nuts (100 calories total, varies based on brand and preparation); 1 oz soy chips (I recommend Revival brand soy chips. Three to four times a week, if desired, you may substitute any 200-calorie food you desire, for example two part-skim mozzarella cheese sticks or 2 oz of chocolate (200 calories).

LUNCH: Garlic Chicken Burrito
  8" whole-wheat tortilla wrap
  3 lettuce leaves
  2 oz chicken
  1 slice tomato
  1 tsp garlic powder
  1 tsp sour cream
  1 oz corn
  1 oz low-fat Mozzarella cheese
  3 oz black beans

MID-AFTERNOON SNACK: Same as mid-morning snack.

DINNER: 2 Crab Cakes, with vegetable.

Family size (serves 4)
  1 egg, beaten
  2 slices of bread, crust removed, broken into crumbs
  1 tbsp seafood seasoning or Old Bay seasoning
  1 tsp Worcestershire sauce
  1 tbsp light mayonnaise
  1/2 tsp baking powder
  1 lb fresh crabmeat

Combine egg, breadcrumbs, seafood seasoning, Worcestershire sauce, mayonnaise and baking powder in a large bowl. Stir in crabmeat. Mix well. Shape mixture into 8 one-half inch thick patties. Broil for 10 minutes without turning.

Eat two crab cakes for a single serving (refrigerate or freeze the rest for later consumption).

Serve with 1 cup of any of the following steamed vegetables: asparagus, broccoli, eggplant, green beans, kale, snow pea pods, or spinach.

1400 CALORIES

Week 3 * Day 4

BREAKFAST: One cup of cereal (see cereal choices) and one cup soy milk or low-fat or skim milk.

MID-MORNING SNACK: Snacks may consist of two of the following choices: banana; apple; pear; 2 cups strawberries (no sugar added); 1.5 cups blueberries (no sugar added); 2 cups raspberries (no sugar added); low-calorie yogurt (100 calories); 1 oz of soy nuts (100 calories total, varies based on brand and preparation); 1 oz soy chips (I recommend Revival brand soy chips. Three to four times a week, if desired, you may substitute any 200-calorie food you desire, for example two part-skim mozzarella cheese sticks or 2 oz of chocolate (200 calories).

LUNCH: Shrimp and Avocado Wrap
   8" whole-wheat tortilla wrap
   4 oz shrimp, fresh or frozen
   1/2 cup avocado, mashed

MID-AFTERNOON SNACK: Same as mid-morning snack.

DINNER: Gingered Beef and Broccoli, with rice.

Family size (serves 4)
   2 cups broccoli (keep stems 1/4 inch)
   1 cup cut snow peas
   1 red pepper, cut in half-inch pieces
   1/2 cup shitake mushrooms
   3/4 lb lean beef, cut for stir-fry
   3 tbsp water
   1.5 tbsp cornstarch
   2 tbsp olive oil
   1 tbsp fresh ginger, minced
   3/4 cup low-sodium soy sauce

Single serving
   1/4 of the above recipe (save the rest in refrigerator).

Add to a bowl the water, cornstarch, and soy sauce. Microwave broccoli, covered, on high power for 3 minutes. Heat non-stick skillet on high. When hot, pour 1 tsp olive oil into pan. Add ginger and beef and stir-fry until beef browns. Add sauce and toss to coat. Remove beef from pan. Add remaining oil. Add broccoli to pan along with peppers, mushrooms and snow peas. Stir-fry for 2 minutes. Return beef with sauce to pan, toss to evenly distribute.

Serve with 4 oz (1/2 cup) of brown rice.

1400 CALORIES

Week 3 * Day 5

BREAKFAST: One cup of cereal (see cereal choices) and one cup soy milk or low-fat or skim milk.

MID-MORNING SNACK: Snacks may consist of two of the following choices: banana; apple; pear; 2 cups strawberries (no sugar added); 1.5 cups blueberries (no sugar added); 2 cups raspberries (no sugar added); low-calorie yogurt (100 calories); 1 oz of soy nuts (100 calories total, varies based on brand and preparation); 1 oz soy chips (I recommend Revival brand soy chips. Three to four times a week, if desired, you may substitute any 200-calorie food you desire, for example two part-skim mozzarella cheese sticks or 2 oz of chocolate (200 calories).

LUNCH: BBQ Pork Wrap
   8" whole-wheat tortilla wrap
   1 tsp onion powder
   2 tsp BBQ sauce
   2 tomato slices
   4 lettuce leaves
   4 oz pork loin

MID-AFTERNOON SNACK: Same as mid-morning snack.

DINNER: Lemon Baked Chicken, with rice and vegetable.

Family size (serves 4)	Single serving
Olive oil cooking spray	Olive oil cooking spray
2 tbsp fresh lemon juice	2 tsp fresh lemon juice
2 tbsp canola oil	2 tsp canola oil
1 clove of garlic, crushed	1/4 clove garlic, crushed
1/2 tsp fresh ground pepper	fresh ground pepper to taste
2-2 1/2 lbs boneless, skinless chicken breasts	6 oz boneless, skinless chicken breast

Preheat oven to 350 degrees. Lightly spray a baking pan or a shallow casserole dish with cooking spray. In a small bowl, combine lemon juice, oil, garlic and pepper. Set aside. Rinse chicken and pat dry. Arrange chicken in prepared pan or dish. Pour lemon mixture over chicken pieces. Cover and bake for 40 minutes, or until tender, basting occasionally. Uncover and bake 10 minutes longer to allow chicken to brown.

Serve with 6 oz (3/4 cup) of cooked brown or wild rice and 1 cup of any of the following steamed vegetables asparagus, broccoli, eggplant, green beans, kale, snow pea pods, or spinach.

1400 CALORIES

Week 3 * Day 6

BREAKFAST: One cup of cereal (see cereal choices) and one cup soy milk or low-fat or skim milk.

MID-MORNING SNACK: Snacks may consist of two of the following choices: banana; apple; pear; 2 cups strawberries (no sugar added); 1.5 cups blueberries (no sugar added); 2 cups raspberries (no sugar added); low-calorie yogurt (100 calories); 1 oz of soy nuts (100 calories total, varies based on brand and preparation); 1 oz soy chips (I recommend Revival brand soy chips. Three to four times a week, if desired, you may substitute any 200-calorie food you desire, for example two part-skim mozzarella cheese sticks or 2 oz of chocolate (200 calories).

LUNCH: Island Wrap
   8" whole-wheat tortilla wrap
   2 lettuce leaves
   4 oz ham
   3 slices tomato
   1 tsp bacon bits
   1 oz mozzarella cheese
   1 oz pineapple
   2 tsp fat-free ranch dressing

MID-AFTERNOON SNACK: Same as mid-morning snack.

DINNER: Spinach Stuffed Sirloin

Family size (serves 4)	Single serving
1 1/2 lb lean sirloin steak, 1" to 1 1/2" thick	6 oz lean sirloin steak, 1" to 1 1/2" thick
1- 10 oz pkg frozen spinach, thawed and drained	4 oz pkg frozen spinach, thawed and drained
2 cloves garlic, crushed	1/2 clove garlic, crushed
cooking oil spray	cooking oil spray
1/4 lb mushrooms, finely chopped	2 oz mushrooms, finely chopped
1/2 cup diced red bell pepper (optional)	2 oz diced red bell pepper (optional)
1 tbsp olive oil	1 tsp olive oil
1/4 cup grated Parmesan cheese	1 oz grated Parmesan cheese

Preheat broiler. Meanwhile, heat oil in small sauté pan until hot but not smoking. Cook garlic, mushroom, and red bell pepper until softened. Add spinach and heat through. Stir in grated Parmesan thoroughly and remove from heat. With a sharp knife, cut pocket in sirloin steak nearly to the edges. Stuff with warm spinach mixture and place on rack in shallow pan. For medium rare, broil for 5 minutes on first side and 3 minutes, approximately, after turning steak over. For other doneness, adjust broiling time accordingly.

Serve with 6 oz (3/4 cup) of cooked brown or wild rice and 1 cup of any of the following steamed vegetables asparagus, broccoli, eggplant, green beans, kale, snow pea pods, or spinach.

1400 CALORIES

Week 3 * Day 7

BREAKFAST: One cup of cereal (see cereal choices) and one cup soy milk or low-fat or skim milk.

MID-MORNING SNACK: Snacks may consist of two of the following choices: banana; apple; pear; 2 cups strawberries (no sugar added); 1.5 cups blueberries (no sugar added); 2 cups raspberries (no sugar added); low-calorie yogurt (100 calories); 1 oz of soy nuts (100 calories total, varies based on brand and preparation); 1 oz soy chips (I recommend Revival brand soy chips. Three to four times a week, if desired, you may substitute any 200-calorie food you desire, for example two part-skim mozzarella cheese sticks or 2 oz of chocolate (200 calories).

LUNCH: BBQ Pork Burrito

8" whole-wheat tortilla wrap	1 oz low-fat mozzarella cheese
3 lettuce leaves	3 oz black beans
2 oz chicken	1 tsp barbeque sauce
3 tomato slices	1 tsp sour cream
1 oz corn	

MID-AFTERNOON SNACK: Same as mid-morning snack.

DINNER: Chicken Manicotti, with rice and vegetable.

Family size (serves 4)	Single serving
3/4 tsp oregano	3/4 tsp oregano
1/2 tsp marjoram	1/2 tsp marjoram
3/4 tsp sweet basil	3/4 tsp sweet basil
1/4 tsp fresh ground pepper	1/4 tsp fresh ground pepper
1- 6 oz can no-salt-added tomato paste	1 - 6 oz can no salt added tomato paste
1 cup water	1 cup water
1 clove garlic, minced	1 clove garlic, minced
4 boneless, skinless chicken breasts, (about 1 lb), fat removed	1 boneless, skinless chicken breast, (6 oz), fat removed
4 oz low-fat cottage cheese, drained	4 oz low-fat cottage cheese, drained
2 oz grated part-skim Mozzarella cheese	2 oz grated part-skim Mozzarella

Preheat oven 350 degrees. In a small bowl, combines the four spices. Mix well. Set aside. In a small saucepan, blend tomato paste, water, and garlic. Add 3/4 of the seasoning mixture to the pan. Bring to a boil. Reduce heat and simmer 10 minutes, stirring occasionally. Meanwhile, rinse chicken and pat dry. Place breast fillets in a plastic bag and pound to 1/4" thickness. Set aside in a small bowl, combine remaining spice mixture with cottage cheese. Spoon mixtures onto centers of chicken breasts, leaving a 1/2 inch edge all around. From narrow end, roll each breast, leaving a 1/2 inch edge all around. Spoon half of the tomato mixture into the bottom of a 10 x 6 inch baking dish. Arrange chicken roll on top, seam side down. Spoon remaining tomato mixture over the chicken rolls. Top with Mozzarella cheese and bake about 45 minutes, or until golden brown.

Serve with 6 oz (3/4 cup) of cooked brown or wild rice and 1 cup of any of the following steamed vegetables: asparagus, broccoli, eggplant, green beans, kale, snow pea pods, or spinach.

1600 CALORIE DIET

Calorie Distribution in 1600 Calorie Diet

Breakfast	250 Calories
Mid-Morning Snack	200 Calories
Lunch	475 Calories
Mid-Afternoon Snack	200 Calories
Dinner	475 Calories

Rules for the North Star Diet

1) Eat breakfast within 20 minutes after waking in the morning. Failure to eat a timely breakfast will decrease your fat-burning capacity, or metabolism. Breakfast choices consist of any high-fiber cereal with non-fat milk fortified with vitamin D and calcium or, preferably, non-fat soy milk fortified with vitamin D and calcium. High-fiber cereals should contain at least 8 grams of fiber in each serving. Recommended high-fiber cereals:

CEREAL	PORTION	CALORIES	FIBER (content)
General Mills Fiber One	1/2 cup	59	14 g
General Mills Fiber One Honey Clusters**	1 1/4 cup	170	14 g
Kellogg's Bran Buds	1/3 cup	80	11 g
Kellogg's All-Bran	1/2 cup	80	10 g
Post or Nabisco			
100% Bran	1/3 cup	80	9 g
Post Raisin Bran	1 cup	190	8 g
Kashi Good Friends	3/4 cup	90	8 g
Kashi Lean Crunch	1 cup	190	8 g
OATMEAL			
Quaker Weight Control	1 serving	160	8 g
TORTILLAS			
Cruz whole-wheat	large 8"	130	11 g
La tortilla factory	large 8"	80	14 g
Mission low carb	6" size	110	11 g

2) Consume mid-morning snacks and mid-afternoon snacks. Both snacks may consist of one (1200 calorie diet) or two (all other diets) of the following choices: banana; apple; pear; 2 cups strawberries (no sugar added); 1.5 cups blueberries (no sugar added); 2 cups raspberries (no sugar added); low-calorie yogurt (100 calories); 1 oz of soy nuts (100 calories total, varies based on brand and preparation); 1 oz soy chips (I recommend Revival brand soy chips). Failure to eat timely mid-morning and mid-afternoon snacks will decrease your fat-burning capacity, or metabolism. Three to four times a week you may substitute any food you desire(100 to 200 calories depending upon meal plan), for example one or two part-skim mozzarella cheese stick(s) or 1-2 oz of chocolate (100-200 calories).

Rules for the North Star Diet, cont'd.

3) Consume 2 liters of fluid a day (approximately 80 ounces). Eighty ounces of fluid is the equivalent of 8 ounces of water per hour for ten hours a day, or two 8-ounce glasses of water with each meal and snack. You may substitute diet soda pop or tea with meals if desired but no fruit juice or regular pop is allowed.

4) Consumption of two cups of green tea, one tea bag per cup, will promote 70 calories of weight loss on a daily basis. A personal favorite is Tazo Zen brand of green tea.

5) Consume dinner 3-4 hours prior to bedtime. If you eat closer to bedtime there is an increased chance the food will be stored and converted into fat while you sleep. If you are still hungry after dinner, you may consume an apple, pear or banana or 1 ounce of lean, grilled protein, e.g. turkey, ham, beef, or fish.

6) The meal plans are to be used as guides. Most individuals only eat 7-10 different foods in a given week. If yo u like certain wraps or dinners and not others, consume those you enjoy the most. I only ask that starting in the second week of the North Star Diet you begin utilizing a whole-wheat wrap/tortilla. (See lunch alternative if you desire to use bread as an alternative). Whole-wheat wraps can often contain as much as 10 –14 g of fiber per serving. They are easy to make. Combine fillings in the center of the tortilla and roll up. I recommend the following whole-wheat tortilla/wraps: Cruz brand whole-wheat tortilla (10 grams of dietary fiber per serving); La Tortilla Factory whol e-wheat, low-carb/low-fat tortillas (large size, 14 grams of fiber); and Carb Down flat bread (14 grams of fiber).

7) Consume daily: a multi-vitamin; 1200 mg of calcium carbonate; 1000 I.U. vitamin D; and 1000-3000 mg of fish oil.

** Personal Favorite

Measurement Conversions

Do not fear the measurements in the following calorie-specific diets. You could weigh each item as described. However, I approximate all food quantities based on the volume of a deck of playing cards.

3 ounces (oz) = the fluid volume of a deck of playing cards.

1 cup = 8 fluid ounces = 2.5 fluid equivalents of a deck of playing cards.

1 ounce (oz) = the fluid equivalent of one-third of a deck of playing cards.

1/2 ounce (oz) = 1 tablespoon (tbsp) = the fluid equivalent of 1/6 of a deck of playing cards.

1600 CALORIES

Week 1 * Day 1

BREAKFAST: One cup of cereal (see cereal choices) and one cup soy milk or low-fat or skim milk.

MID-MORNING SNACK: Snacks may consist of two of the following choices: banana; apple; pear; 2 cups strawberries (no sugar added); 1.5 cups blueberries (no sugar added); 2 cups raspberries (no sugar added); low-calorie yogurt (100 calories); 1 oz of soy nuts (100 calories total, varies based on brand and preparation); 1 oz soy chips (I recommend Revival brand soy chips. Three to four times a week, if desired, you may substitute any 200-calorie food you desire, for example two part-skim mozzarella cheese sticks or 2 oz of chocolate (200 calories).

LUNCH: Mediterranean Wrap
  8" tortilla wrap
  6 oz turkey, roasted or sl iced, skinless white meat
  4 lettuce leaves
  2 oz cucumber strips
  1 tsp red pepper flakes
  1 oz feta cheese
  2 tsp fat-free red wine vinegar

MID-AFTERNOON SNACK: Same as mid-morning snack.

DINNER: Crispy Baked Chicken, with rice and vegetable.

Family size (4 servings)	Single serving
2-2.5 lbs boneless, skinless chicken breasts	8 oz boneless, skinless chicken breast
1 cup skim milk	1/4 cup skim milk
1 cup cornflake crumbs	1/4 cup cornflake crumbs
1 tsp rosemary	1 pinch rosemary
1 tsp fresh ground black pepper	1 pinch fresh ground black pepper
Pam cooking oil spray	Pam cooking oil spray or olive oil spray

Preheat oven to 350 degrees. Cover a baking dish with foil and spray lightly with cooking oil spray. Rinse chicken and pat dry. Set aside. Pour milk into a shallow bowl. Combine cornflake crumbs, rosemary, and pepper in another shallow bowl. Dip chicken first into milk and then into crumb mixture. Allow to stand briefly so coating will adhere. Arrange chicken in prepared pan so pieces do not touch. Bake 40 minutes or until done. Crumbs will form a crisp "skin".

Serve with 3/4 cup of cooked wild or brown rice and 1 cup of any of the following steamed vegetables: asparagus, broccoli, eggplant, green beans, kale, snow pea pods, or spinach.

1600 CALORIES

Week 1 * Day 2

BREAKFAST: One cup of cereal (see cereal choices) and one cup soy milk or low-fat or skim milk.

MID-MORNING SNACK: Snacks may consist of two of the following choices: banana; apple; pear; 2 cups strawberries (no sugar added); 1.5 cups blueberries (no sugar added); 2 cups raspberries (no sugar added); low-calorie yogurt (100 calories); 1 oz of soy nuts (100 calories total, varies based on brand and preparation); 1 oz soy chips (I recommend Revival brand soy chips. Three to four times a week, if desired, you may substitute any 200-calorie food you desire, for example two part-skim mozzarella cheese sticks or 2 oz of chocolate (200 calories).

LUNCH: Beef Taquito Wrap
   8" tortilla wrap
   4 oz round steak, trimmed
   1 oz mozzarella low-fat cheese
   2 tsp salsa

MID-AFTERNOON SNACK: Same as mid-morning snack.

DINNER: Scallops Oriental, with rice and vegetable.

Family size (4 servings)	Single serving
cooking oil spray (preferably olive oil)	cooking oil spray (preferably olive oil)
1 1/2 lb fresh or frozen scallops	6 oz of fresh or frozen scallops
1/8 cup of honey	2 tsp honey
1/8 cup mustard	2 tsp mustard
1/2 tsp curry powder	pinch curry powder
1/2 tsp lemon juice	1/8 tsp lemon juice

Preheat broiler. Lightly spray baking pan with cooking spray. Rinse scallops and drain. Place in a baking pan. In a saucepan, combine remaining ingredients. Brush scallops with sauce. Broil 4 inches from heat for 5-8 minutes or until browned.

Serve with 3/4 cup of cooked wild or brown rice and 1 cup of any of the following steamed vegetables: asparagus, broccoli, eggplant, green beans, kale, snow pea pods, or spinach.

1600 CALORIES

Week 1 * Day 3

BREAKFAST: One cup of cereal (see cereal choices) and one cup soy milk or low-fat or skim milk.

MID-MORNING SNACK: Snacks may consist of two of the following choices: banana; apple; pear; 2 cups strawberries (no sugar added); 1.5 cups blueberries (no sugar added); 2 cups raspberries (no sugar added); low-calorie yogurt (100 calories); 1 oz of soy nuts (100 calories total, varies based on brand and preparation); 1 oz soy chips (I recommend Revival brand soy chips. Three to four times a week, if desired, you may substitute any 200-calorie food you desire, for example two part-skim mozzarella cheese sticks or 2 oz of chocolate (200 calories).

LUNCH: Tuna Mayo Wrap
   8" tortilla wrap
   2 oz low-fat mayonnaise
   8 oz tuna
   1/4 rib celery

MID-AFTERNOON SNACK: Same as mid-morning snack.

DINNER: Tomato, Mushroom, and Jack Cheese Omelet, with vegetable and baked potato.

Single Serving
   Cooking oil spray (olive oil preferable)
   4 eggs or egg substitute equivalent
   1/4 cup seeded, chopped tomato
   1/2 oz shredded, low-fat Monterey -Jack cheese
   1/4 cup mushrooms
   1 tsp chopped cilantro or parsley
   Hot pepper sauce (optional)

Spray skillet with cooking oil, or use non-stick frying pan. Place pan over medium high heat. In a small bowl, place eggs or egg substitute . Beat and pour mixture into pan. Stir eggs in a circular motion. Do not scrape bottom of pan. When the omelet is almost cooked, add fillings. Fold omelet over with a fork while holding the pan at 45-degree angle. Roll omelet onto plate and serve.

Serve with 1 medium (7 oz) baked potato with 1 tsp soft canola margarine, and 1 cup of any of the following steamed vegetables: asparagus, broccoli, eggplant, green beans, kale, snow pea pods, or spinach.

1600 CALORIES

Week 1 * Day 4

BREAKFAST: One cup of cereal (see cereal choices) and one cup soy milk or low-fat or skim milk.

MID-MORNING SNACK: Snacks may consist of two of the following choices: banana; apple; pear; 2 cups strawberries (no sugar added); 1.5 cups blueberries (no sugar added); 2 cups raspberries (no sugar added); low-calorie yogurt (100 calories); 1 oz of soy nuts (100 calories total, varies based on brand and preparation); 1 oz soy chips (I recommend Revival brand soy chips. Three to four times a week, if desired, you may substitute any 200-calorie food you desire, for example two part-skim mozzarella cheese sticks or 2 oz of chocolate (200 calories).

LUNCH: Beef Wrap
   8"whole-wheat tortilla wrap
   6 oz broiled, trimmed round steak
   1/2 cup raw or broiled mushrooms
   2 tsp Worcestershire sauce
   1 tsp soy sauce

MID-AFTERNOON SNACK: Same as mid-morning snack.

DINNER: Mustard-Crusted Pork, with rice and vegetable.

Serving for two
   2 tsp soy or tofu flour (available at most health food stores)
   1 tsp mustard powder
   1/2 tsp pepper
   1/4 cup olive oil
   1 lb boneless, center-cut pork chops, cut against the grain into 3" strips, about 3/8 " thick

Single serving
   2 tsp soy or tofu flour (available at most health food stores)
   1 tsp mustard powder
   1/2 tsp pepper
   1/4 cup olive oil
   8 oz boneless, center-cut pork chops, cut against the grain into 3" strips, about 3/8 " thick

Combine the flour, mustard powder, and pepper in a bowl and mix well. Dust the pork with the flour mixture. Heat 2 tbs oil over medium heat until hot but not smoking. Add half the pork and brown for five minutes on each side, or until cooked through. Repeat with the remaining pork. Sprinkle with seasoning. Remove from heat and serve immediately.

Serve with 3/4 cup of cooked wild or brown rice and 1 cup of any of the following steamed vegetables: asparagus, broccoli, eggplant, green beans, kale, snow pea pods, or spinach.

1600 CALORIES

Week 1 * Day 5

BREAKFAST: One cup of cereal (see cereal choices) and one cup soy milk or low-fat or skim milk.

MID-MORNING SNACK: Snacks may consist of two of the following choices: banana; apple; pear; 2 cups strawberries (no sugar added); 1.5 cups blueberries (no sugar added); 2 cups raspberries (no sugar added); low-calorie yogurt (100 calories); 1 oz of soy nuts (100 calories total, varies based on brand and preparation); 1 oz soy chips (I recommend Revival brand soy chips. Three to four times a week, if desired, you may substitute any 200-calorie food you desire, for example two part-skim mozzarella cheese sticks or 2 oz of chocolate (200 calories).

LUNCH: Turkey Vegetable Wraps
   8" whole-wheat tortilla wrap
   6 oz turkey, roasted or sl iced, skinless white meat
   1 oz corn, canned in water
   1 oz red pepper
   1 oz green onion
   2 tsp fat-free, light ranch dressing

MID-AFTERNOON SNACK: Same as mid-morning snack.

DINNER: Fish Fillets with Asparagus, with rice and vegetable.

Family size (serves four)	Single serving
Cooking oil spray (preferably olive oil)	Cooking oil spray (preferably olive oil
4 - 5 oz mild, white fish fillets (Haddock, cod, etc.)	1 - 5 oz mild, white fish fillet (Haddock, cod, etc.)
1/2 tsp ground black pepper	1/4 tsp ground black pepper
2 tbsp unsalted butter	1 tbsp unsalted butter
12 stalks cooked asparagus	3 stalks cooked asparagus
1/3 cup tangy sour cream	1/3 cup tangy sour cream
1/3 cup plain low-fat yogurt	1/3 cup plain low-fat yogurt
2 tsp minced chives	1 tsp minced chives
2 tsp horseradish	1 tsp horseradish
1 egg white	1 egg white
2 tsp chopped parsley	1 tsp chopped parsley

Preheat broiler. Lightly spray broiler pan with cooking spray. Rinse fish and pat dry. Season fish with pepper and lemon juice and brush with margarine. Place on broiler pan and broil about 8 minutes or until fish almost flakes. Remove from oven and top each filet with 3 stalks of asparagus. In a small bowl, combine sour cream, yogurt, chives, horseradish, and dill weed. In another bowl, beat egg whites until stiff peaks form; fold into sour cream mixture. Spread mixture over each fillet to cover fish and asparagus. Return to broiler and broil 1-2 minutes, or until golden brown. Sprinkle with parsley.

Serve with 3/4 cup of cooked wild or brown rice and 1 cup of any of the following steamed vegetables: asparagus, broccoli, eggplant, green beans, kale, snow pea pods, or spinach.

1600 CALORIES

Week 1 * Day 6

BREAKFAST: One cup of cereal (see cereal choices) and one cup soy milk or low-fat or skim milk.

MID-MORNING SNACK: Snacks may consist of two of the following choices: banana; apple; pear; 2 cups strawberries (no sugar added); 1.5 cups blueberries (no sugar added); 2 cups raspberries (no sugar added); low-calorie yogurt (100 calories); 1 oz of soy nuts (100 calories total, varies based on brand and preparation); 1 oz soy chips (I recommend Revival brand soy chips. Three to four times a week, if desired, you may substitute any 200-calorie food you desire, for example two part-skim mozzarella cheese sticks or 2 oz of chocolate (200 calories).

LUNCH: California Chicken Wrap
   8" whole-wheat tortilla wrap
   5 oz grilled white chicken
   2 tsp guacamole
   3 tomato slices
   3 lettuce leaves
   1 tsp bacon bits

MID-AFTERNOON SNACK: Same as mid-morning snack.

DINNER: Feta Burgers, with rice and steamed vegetable.

Family size (serves 4)
   cooking oil spray, preferably olive oil
   1 lb ground sirloin or ground round
   1/4 cup crumbled feta cheese
   1/4 cup finely chopped black olives
   1/2 tsp salt
   1/2 tsp. pepper

Single serving
   6 oz ground sirloin or ground round
   1 oz feta cheese
   1 oz finely chopped black olives
   salt and pepper to taste

Heat pan sprayed with cooking spray. Mix remaining ingredients and shape into four patties (one for single serving). Sauté patties at medium high heat for 5 minutes on each side or to desired doneness.

Serve with 3/4 cup of cooked wild or brown rice and 1 cup of any of the following steamed vegetables: asparagus, broccoli, eggplant, green beans, kale, snow pea pods, or spinach.

1600 CALORIES

Week 1 * Day 7

BREAKFAST: One cup of cereal (see cereal choices) and one cup soy milk or low-fat or skim milk.

MID-MORNING SNACK: Snacks may consist of two of the following choices: banana; apple; pear; 2 cups strawberries (no sugar added); 1.5 cups blueberries (no sugar added); 2 cups raspberries (no sugar added); low-calorie yogurt (100 calories); 1 oz of soy nuts (100 calories total, varies based on brand and preparation); 1 oz soy chips (I recommend Revival brand soy chips. Three to four times a week, if desired, you may substitute any 200-calorie food you desire, for example two part-skim mozzarella cheese sticks or 2 oz of chocolate (200 calories).

LUNCH: Ham Club Wrap
   8" tortilla wrap
   4 oz ham
   3 slices tomato
   3 lettuce leaves
   1 tsp bacon bits
   1 tsp light Italian dressing
   1 oz low-fat Mozzarella cheese

MID-AFTERNOON SNACK: Same as mid-morning snack.

DINNER: Lemon Baked Chicken, with rice and steamed vegetable.

Family size (serves 4)	Single serving
Olive oil cooking spray	olive oil cooking spray
2 tsp fresh lemon juice	1 tsp fresh lemon juice
2 tsp low fat margarine or safflower oil	1 tsp low-fat margarine or safflower oil
1 clove garlic, crushed	1/4 clove garlic, crushed
1/2 tsp fresh ground black pepper	1/8 tsp fresh ground black pepper
2 lbs of boneless, skinless chicken breast.	8 oz boneless, skinless chicken breast

Preheat oven to 350 degrees. Lightly spray a baking pan or a shallow casserole dish with cooking spray. In a small bowl, combine lemon juice, oil, garlic and pepper. Set aside. Rinse chicken and pat dry. Arrange chicken in prepared pan or dish. Pour lemon mixture over chicken pieces. Cover and bake 40 minutes or until tender, basting occasionally. Uncover and bake 10 minutes longer to allow chicken to brown.

Serve with 3/4 cup of cooked wild or brown rice and 1 cup of any of the following steamed vegetables: asparagus, broccoli, eggplant, green beans, kale, snow pea pods, or spinach.

1600 CALORIES

Week 2 * Day 1

BREAKFAST: One cup of cereal (see cereal choices) and one cup soy milk or low-fat or skim milk.

MID-MORNING SNACK: Snacks may consist of two of the following choices: banana; apple; pear; 2 cups strawberries (no sugar added); 1.5 cups blueberries (no sugar added); 2 cups raspberries (no sugar added); low-calorie yogurt (100 calories); 1 oz of soy nuts (100 calories total, varies based on brand and preparation); 1 oz soy chips (I recommend Revival brand soy chips. Three to four times a week, if desired, you may substitute any 200-calorie food you desire, for example two part-skim mozzarella cheese sticks or 2 oz of chocolate (200 calories).

LUNCH: Chicken with zucchini and roasted pepper wrap
    8" whole-wheat tortilla wrap
    4 oz broiled white chicken meat
    3-4 oz zucchini
    2 oz pickled sweet peppers
    1 oz part-skim, reduced-fat mozzarella cheese

MID-AFTERNOON SNACK: Same as mid-morning snack.

DINNER: Pineapple and Shrimp, with rice and vegetable

Family size (Serves 4)
    1 clove garlic, crushed
    2 tbsp canola margarine
    1/4 cup honey
    1 tbsp sweet chili sauce
    1 tbsp soy sauce
    1 whole pineapple, or 20 oz canned in water or light syrup
    2 lbs of shrimp, fresh or frozen, peeled and de-veined

Single serving
    1 tsp garlic powder or 1/4 clove of garlic, crushed
    2 tsp canola margarine
    1 oz honey
    1 tsp sweet chili sauce
    1 tsp soy sauce
    6 oz fresh pineapple, or 6 oz canned in water or light syrup
    8 oz shrimp, fresh or frozen, peeled and de-veined

Combine first five ingredients in a bowl. Brush shrimp with the mixture. Grill at high temperature for 5 minutes. Add pineapple.

Serve with 3/4 cup of cooked wild or brown rice and 1 cup of any of the following steamed vegetables: asparagus, broccoli, eggplant, greenbeans, kale, snowpeapods, or spinach.

1600 CALORIES

Week 2 * Day 2

BREAKFAST: One cup of cereal (see cereal choices) and one cup soy milk or low-fat or skim milk.

MID-MORNING SNACK: Snacks may consist of two of the following choices: banana; apple; pear; 2 cups strawberries (no sugar added); 1.5 cups blueberries (no sugar added); 2 cups raspberries (no sugar added); low-calorie yogurt (100 calories); 1 oz of soy nuts (100 calories total, varies based on brand and preparation); 1 oz soy chips (I recommend Revival brand soy chips. Three to four times a week, if desired, you may substitute any 200-calorie food you desire, for example two part-skim mozzarella cheese sticks or 2 oz of chocolate (200 calories).

LUNCH: Santa Fe Steak Burrito
   8" whole-wheat tortilla wrap
   2 oz steak
   1 oz corn
   3 oz black beans
   1 tsp sour cream
   3 lettuce leaves
   3 tomato slices
   1 oz low-fat mozzarella cheese
   2 tsp salsa

MID-AFTERNOON SNACK: Same as mid-morning snack.

DINNER: Turkey Burgers, with wild rice and steamed vegetable.

Family size (serves 4)	Single serving
1 1/2 lb ground turkey (90% lean), thawed	6 oz ground turkey (90% lean), thawed
1/4 cup onions, or powdered onion flakes	1 oz onions, or powdered onion flakes
2 tbsp green peppers	2 tsp green peppers
1 tbsp Worcestershire Sauce	1 tsp Worcestershire sauce
2 tbsp ketchup	1 tsp ketchup
1/4 tsp black pepper	1/8 tsp black pepper
lettuce leaves	lettuce leaves
tomato slices	tomato slices
4 whole-wheat pita pockets	1 whole-wheat pita pocket

Form ground turkey and seasonings into patties. Grill or broil for 5 minutes per side, or until done. Top patties with lettuce and tomato and place in pita pocket.

Serve with 4 oz (1/2 cup) of cooked brown or wild rice and 1 cup of any of the following steamed vegetables: asparagus, broccoli, eggplant, green beans, kale, snow pea pods, or spinach.

1600 CALORIES

Week 2 *Day 3

BREAKFAST: One cup of cereal (see cereal choices) and one cup soy milk or low-fat or skim milk.

MID-MORNING SNACK: Snacks may consist of two of the following choices: banana; apple; pear; 2 cups strawberries (no sugar added); 1.5 cups blueberries (no sugar added); 2 cups raspberries (no sugar added); low-calorie yogurt (100 calories); 1 oz of soy nuts (100 calories total, varies based on brand and preparation); 1 oz soy chips (I recommend Revival brand soy chips. Three to four times a week, if desired, you may substitute any 200-calorie food you desire, for example two part-skim mozzarella cheese sticks or 2 oz of chocolate (200 calories).

LUNCH: Tasty Turkey Wrap
  8" whole-wheat tortilla wrap
  onion powder to taste
  6 oz turkey
  2 tsp sliced olives
  1 oz mozzarella low-fat cheese
  2 tsp fat-free mayo
  3 lettuce leaves
  1 tsp mustard
  3 slices tomato

MID-AFTERNOON SNACK: Same as mid-morning snack.

DINNER: Chicken with Mushrooms, with baked potato and vegetable.

Family size (serves 4)	Single serving
4 - 8 oz chicken breasts, skinless	8 oz chicken breast, skinless
20 oz button mushrooms	5 oz button mushrooms
1/2 tsp pepper	1/2 tsp pepper
2 tbsp olive oil	1 garlic clove
4 garlic cloves	1 tbsp olive oil
juice of 1/2 lemon	juice of 1/4 lemon
1 cup dry white wine	1/2 cup dry white wine
pinch of dried hot red pepper flakes	pinch of dried hot red pepper flakes

Grill chicken, set aside. Heat oil in a heavy skillet over medium heat. Add the garlic, lemon juice, wine, pepper, and red pepper flakes. Bring to a boil. Lower heat and add mushrooms. Simmer and stir frequently for 5–6 minutes. Add pre-grilled chicken.

Serve with 1 medium (7 oz) baked potato with 1 tsp soft canola margarine, and 1 cup of any of the following steamed vegetables: asparagus, broccoli, eggplant, greenbeans, kale, snow pea pods, or spinach.

1600 CALORIES

Week 2 * Day 4

BREAKFAST: One cup of cereal (see cereal choices) and one cup soy milk or low-fat or skim milk.

MID-MORNING SNACK: Snacks may consist of two of the following choices: banana; apple; pear; 2 cups strawberries (no sugar added); 1.5 cups blueberries (no sugar added); 2 cups raspberries (no sugar added); low-calorie yogurt (100 calories); 1 oz of soy nuts (100 calories total, varies based on brand and preparation); 1 oz soy chips (I recommend Revival brand soy chips. Three to four times a week, if desired, you may substitute any 200-calorie food you desire, for example two part-skim mozzarella cheese sticks or 2 oz of chocolate (200 calories).

LUNCH: Greek Wrap
   8" whole-wheat tortilla wrap
   6 oz grilled chicken breast, no skin
   1 oz feta cheese (reduced-fat)
   4 lettuce leaves
   2-3 tomato slices
   2 tsp low-calorie vinaigrette dressing

MID-AFTERNOON SNACK: Same as mid-morning snack.

DINNER: Pork with Green Chile and Cheese, and rice and vegetable.

Family size (serves 4)	Single serving
2 lbs boneless, center-cut loin pork chops or sirloin pork steaks (fat removed)	8 oz boneless, center cut loin pork chops or sirloin pork steaks (fat removed)
2 tbsp olive oil	1 tsp olive oil
1/2 cup green chili salsa	2 oz green chili salsa
3/4 cup low-fat cheese, shredded (feta, Muenster, cheddar, or mozzarella)	2 oz low-fat cheese, shredded (feta, Muenster, cheddar, or mozzarella)

Heat oil in pan over medium heat until hot but not smoking. Add pork to pan and brown for 3-5 minutes. Turn heat to low, add 1/2 cup water, and cover pan. Cook for 20-25 minutes or until water is nearly evaporated. Pour salsa over pork, covering evenly. Sprinkle with shredded cheese, cover and cook for additional 3 to 5 minutes or until salsa is heated and cheese is melted.

Serve immediately with 6 oz (3/4 cup) of cooked brown or wild rice and 1 cup of any of the following steamed vegetables: asparagus, broccoli, eggplant, green beans, kale, snow pea pods, or spinach.

1600 CALORIES

Week 2 * Day 5

BREAKFAST: One cup of cereal (see cereal choices) and one cup soy milk or low-fat or skim milk.

MID-MORNING SNACK: Snacks may consist of two of the following choices: banana; apple; pear; 2 cups strawberries (no sugar added); 1.5 cups blueberries (no sugar added); 2 cups raspberries (no sugar added); low-calorie yogurt (100 calories); 1 oz of soy nuts (100 calories total, varies based on brand and preparation); 1 oz soy chips (I recommend Revival brand soy chips. Three to four times a week, if desired, you may substitute any 200-calorie food you desire, for example two part-skim mozzarella cheese sticks or 2 oz of chocolate (200 calories).

LUNCH: Bean and Cheese Burrito
   8" whole-wheat tortilla wrap
   3 oz reduced-fat cheddar cheese
   7 oz black beans
   3 lettuce leaves

Heat, if desired, in microwave or toaster oven.

MID-AFTERNOON SNACK: Same as mid-morning snack.

DINNER: Tandoori Chicken, with rice and vegetable.

Family Size (serves 4)
   4 - 8 oz chicken breasts, skinless
   3 tsp tandoori spice mix
   1 tsp fresh ginger, grated
   1 1/2 cups plain, non-fat yogurt

Single serving
   1 - 8 oz chicken breast, skinless
   1 tsp tandoori spice mix
   1/3 tsp fresh ginger, grated
   1/2 cups plain, non-fat yogurt

Mix yogurt, tandoori spice, cumin and ginger in a bowl. Brush mixture onto chicken breasts. Grill on high for 2 minutes on each side. Reduce heat and cook 5 minutes longer on each side, basting while cooking.

Serve with 6 oz (3/4 cup) of cooked brown or wild rice and 1 cup of any of the following steamed vegetables: asparagus, broccoli, eggplant, green beans, kale, snow pea pods, or spinach.

1600 CALORIES

Week 2 * Day 6

BREAKFAST: One cup of cereal (see cereal choices) and one cup soy milk or low-fat or skim milk.

MID-MORNING SNACK: Snacks may consist of two of the following choices: banana; apple; pear; 2 cups strawberries (no sugar added); 1.5 cups blueberries (no sugar added); 2 cups raspberries (no sugar added); low-calorie yogurt (100 calories); 1 oz of soy nuts (100 calories total, varies based on brand and preparation); 1 oz soy chips (I recommend Revival brand soy chips.Three to four times a week, if desired, you may substitute any 200-calorie food you desire, for example two part-skim mozzarella cheese sticks or 2 oz of chocolate (200 calories).

LUNCH: Chicken Taquito
  8" whole-wheat tortilla wrap
  1 oz low-fat cheddar cheese
  6 oz white chicken meat
  2 tsp salsa

Heat in microwave or in toaster oven

MID-AFTERNOON SNACK: Same as mid-morning snack.

DINNER: Shrimp Scampi, wi th rice and vegetable.

Family size (serves 4)	Single serving
4 tbsp butter (unsalted)	1 tbsp butter (unsalted)
4 tbsp olive oil	1 tbsp olive oil
6 large cloves garlic, minced	1-2 large cloves garlic minced
1/2 cup chopped, fresh **flat-leaf** parsley	2 oz or 1/8 cup chopped, fresh **flat-leaf** parsley
juice of 1 lemon	juice of 1/4 lemon
1 cup dry white wine	2 oz or 1/4 cup of dry white wine
2 pinches dried, hot red pepper **flakes**	1 pinch of dried, hot red pepper **flakes**
salt and black pepper to taste.	salt and black pepper to taste
2 1/2 lbs large shrimp, shelled and de-veined, frozen or fresh	10 oz large shrimp, shelled and de-veined, frozen or fresh

Heat the butter and oil in a skillet over medium heat until the foam subsides. Add the garlic, parsley, lemon juice, wine, pepper **flakes,** salt and pepper. Bring to a boil, lower the heat, and simmer for 3 minutes. Add the shrimp to the skillet and cook, stirring frequently, for 5 to 6 minutes until the shrimp are pink. Remove from heat. Place the shrimp on a serving plate and pour the sauce from the skillet over them.

Serve immediately with 6 oz (3/4cup) of cooked brown or wild rice and 1 cup of any of the following steamed vegetables: asparagus, broccoli, eggplant, green beans, kale, snow pea pods, or spinach.

1600 CALORIES

Week 2 * Day 7

BREAKFAST: One cup of cereal (see cereal choices) and one cup soy milk or low-fat or skim milk.

MID-MORNING SNACK: Snacks may consist of two of the following choices: banana; apple; pear; 2 cups strawberries (no sugar added); 1.5 cups blueberries (no sugar added); 2 cups raspberries (no sugar added); low-calorie yogurt (100 calories); 1 oz of soy nuts (100 calories total, varies based on brand and preparation); 1 oz soy chips (I recommend Revival brand soy chips. Three to four times a week, if desired, you may substitute any 200-calorie food you desire, for example two part-skim mozzarella cheese sticks or 2 oz of chocolate (200 calories).

LUNCH: Vegetarian Greek Wrap
  8" whole-wheat tortilla wrap
  1 oz black olives
  2 tbsp guacamole
  2 oz cucumber
  3 slices tomato
  1 oz feta cheese (reduced-fat)
  4 oz hummus

MID-AFTERNOON SNACK: Same as mid-morning snack.

DINNER: Grilled Spicy Chicken Breast Fillets, with rice and vegetable.

Family size (Serves 4)	Single serving
1 small clove garlic, crushed	1 small clove garlic, crushed
1 small onion, finely chopped	1 small onion, finely chopped
2-3 tbsp lime juice	2-3 tbsp lime juice
2 tbsp olive oil	2 tbsp olive oil
1/2 tsp chili powder	1/2 tsp chili powder
fresh ground pepper to taste	fresh ground pepper to taste
4 - 8 oz boneless, skinless chicken breasts	1 - 8 oz boneless, skinless chicken breast

In a small bowl, combine ingredients. Coat chicken pieces thoroughly. On preheated grill or in broiler, cook chicken, turning once, 6-7 minutes, or until done.

Serve with 6 oz (3/4 cup) of cooked brown or wild rice and 1 cup of any of the following steamed vegetables: asparagus, broccoli, eggplant, green beans, kale, snow pea pods, or spinach.

1600 CALORIES

Week 3 * Day 1

BREAKFAST: One cup of cereal (see cereal choices) and one cup soy milk or low-fat or skim milk.

MID-MORNING SNACK: Snacks may consist of two of the following choices: banana; apple; pear; 2 cups strawberries (no sugar added); 1.5 cups blueberries (no sugar added); 2 cups raspberries (no sugar added); low-calorie yogurt (100 calories); 1 oz of soy nuts (100 calories total, varies based on brand and preparation); 1 oz soy chips (I recommend Revival brand soy chips. Three to four times a week, if desired, you may substitute any 200-calorie food you desire, for example two part-skim mozzarella cheese sticks or 2 oz of chocolate (200 calories).

LUNCH: Ham and Cheese Wrap
   8" whole-wheat tortilla wrap
   6 oz Healthy Choice ham (low-fat ham)
   2 tsp mustard
   1 oz cheddar cheese (low-fat if available)

MID-AFTERNOON SNACK: Same as mid-morning snack.

DINNER: Caribbean Grilled Tuna, with rice and vegetable.

Family size (serves 4)
   cooking oil spray
   4 – 8 oz tuna steaks
   1 tbsp lime and lemon juice
   3 tbsp olive oil
   1 tbsp of Caribbean Jerk Seasoning or Old Bay crab spice mixture

Single serving
   cooking oil spray
   1 - 8 oz tuna steak
   1 tsp lime and lemon juice
   1 tbsp olive oil
   1 tsp Caribbean Jerk Seasoning or Old Bay crab spice mixture

Mix together juice, oil, and seasonings. Brush mixture on to tuna steaks. Spray pan with olive oil cooking spray. Preheat grill or broiler pan. Place tuna on broiler. Grill or broil 5 minutes per side or until fish flakes with a fork.

Serve with 1 cup of cooked brown or wild rice and 1 cup of any of the following steamed vegetables: asparagus, broccoli, eggplant, green beans, kale, snow pea pods, or spinach.

1600 CALORIES

Week 3 * Day 2

BREAKFAST: One cup of cereal (see cereal choices) and one cup soy milk or low-fat or skim milk.

MID-MORNING SNACK: Snacks may consist of two of the following choices: banana; apple; pear; 2 cups strawberries (no sugar added); 1.5 cups blueberries (no sugar added); 2 cups raspberries (no sugar added); low-calorie yogurt (100 calories); 1 oz of soy nuts (100 calories total, varies based on brand and preparation); 1 oz soy chips (I recommend Revival brand soy chips. Three to four times a week, if desired, you may substitute any 200-calorie food you desire, for example two part-skim mozzarella cheese sticks or 2 oz of chocolate (200 calories).

LUNCH: Bar-B-Q Chicken Quesadilla
   8" whole-wheat tortilla wrap
   5 oz chicken
   2 tsp BBQ sauce
   1 1/2 oz reduced-fat cheddar cheese

MID-AFTERNOON SNACK: Same as mid-morning snack.

DINNER: Lemon Pepper Beef Steak, with baked potato and vegetable.

Family size (serves 4)
   1 3/4 lbs of lean beef steak, sirloin tip or round
   1 tbsp olive oil
   2 garlic cloves, crushed
   2 tsp oregano
   1/2 tsp lemon pepper salt

Single serving
   7 oz lean beef steak, sirloin tip or round
   1 tsp olive oil
   1 garlic clove, crushed
   1 tsp oregano
   1/4 tsp lemon pepper salt

Combine seasoning ingredients in a bowl. Brush seasonings on steak. Broil steak until desired doneness.

Serve with 1 small (6 oz) baked potato, with 1 tsp soft canola margarine, and 1 cup of any of the following steamed vegetables: asparagus, broccoli, eggplant, green beans, kale, snow pea pods, or spinach.

1600 CALORIES

Week 3 * Day 3

BREAKFAST: One cup of cereal (see cereal choices) and one cup soy milk or low-fat or skim milk.

MID-MORNING SNACK: Snacks may consist of two of the following choices: banana; apple; pear; 2 cups strawberries (no sugar added); 1.5 cups blueberries (no sugar added); 2 cups raspberries (no sugar added); low-calorie yogurt (100 calories); 1 oz of soy nuts (100 calories total, varies based on brand and preparation); 1 oz soy chips (I recommend Revival brand soy chips. Three to four times a week, if desired, you may substitute any 200-calorie food you desire, for example two part-skim mozzarella cheese sticks or 2 oz of chocolate (200 calories).

LUNCH: Garlic Chicken Burrito
   8" whole-wheat tortilla wrap
   3 lettuce leaves
   4 oz chicken
   1 slice tomato
   1 tsp garlic powder
   1 tsp sour cream
   1 oz corn
   1 oz low-fat mozzarella cheese
   3 oz black beans

MID-AFTERNOON SNACK: Same as mid-morning snack.

DINNER: 2 Crab Cakes, with vegetable.

Family size (serves 4)
   1 egg, beaten
   2 slices of bread, crust removed, broken into crumbs
   1 tbsp seafood seasoning or Old Bay seasoning
   1 tsp Worcestershire sauce
   1 tbsp light mayonnaise
   1/2 tsp baking powder
   1 lb fresh crabmeat

Combine egg, breadcrumbs, seafood seasoning, Worcestershire sauce, mayonnaise and baking powder in a large bowl. Stir in crabmeat. Mix well. Shape mixture into 8 one-half inch thick patties. Broil for 10 minutes without turning.

Eat two crab cakes for a single serving (refrigerate or freeze the rest for later consumption) and serve with 1 cup of any of the following steamed vegetables: asparagus, broccoli, eggplant, green beans, kale, snow pea pods, or spinach.

1600 CALORIES

Week 3 * Day 4

BREAKFAST: One cup of cereal (see cereal choices) and one cup soy milk or low-fat or skim milk.

MID-MORNING SNACK: Snacks may consist of two of the following choices: banana; apple; pear; 2 cups strawberries (no sugar added); 1.5 cups blueberries (no sugar added); 2 cups raspberries (no sugar added); low-calorie yogurt (100 calories); 1 oz of soy nuts (100 calories total, varies based on brand and preparation); 1 oz soy chips (I recommend Revival brand soy chips. Three to four times a week, if desired, you may substitute any 200-calorie food you desire, for example two part-skim mozzarella cheese sticks or 2 oz of chocolate (200 calories).

LUNCH: Shrimp and Avocado Wrap
    8" whole-wheat tortilla wrap
    6 oz shrimp, fresh or frozen
    1/2 cup, mashed

MID-AFTERNOON SNACK: Same as mid-morning snack.

DINNER: Gingered Beef and Broccoli, with rice.

Family size (serves 4)
    2 cups broccoli (keep stems 1/4 inch)
    1 cup cut snow peas
    1 red pepper, cut in half-inch pieces
    1/2 cup shitake mushrooms
    1 1/4 lb lean beef, cut for stir-fry
    3 tbsp water
    1 1/2 tbsp cornstarch
    2 tbsp olive oil
    1 tbsp fresh ginger, minced
    3/4 cup low-sodium soy sauce

Single serving
    1/4 of the above recipe (save the rest in refrigerator).

Add to a bowl the water, cornstarch, and soy sauce. Microwave broccoli, covered, on high power for 3 minutes. Heat non-stick skillet on high. When hot, pour 1 tsp olive oil into pan. Add ginger and beef and stir fry until beef browns. Add sauce and toss to coat. Remove beef from pan. Add remaining oil. Add broccoli to pan along with peppers, mushrooms and snow peas. Stir fry for 2 minutes. Return beef with sauce to pan, toss to evenly distribute.

Serve with 4 oz (1/2 cup) of brown rice.

1600 CALORIES

Week 3 * Day 5

BREAKFAST: One cup of cereal (see cereal choices) and one cup soy milk or low-fat or skim milk.

MID-MORNING SNACK: Snacks may consist of two of the following choices: banana; apple; pear; 2 cups strawberries (no sugar added); 1.5 cups blueberries (no sugar added); 2 cups raspberries (no sugar added); low-calorie yogurt (100 calories); 1 oz of soy nuts (100 calories total, varies based on brand and preparation); 1 oz soy chips (I recommend Revival brand soy chips. Three to four times a week, if desired, you may substitute any 200-calorie food you desire, for example two part-skim mozzarella cheese sticks or 2 oz of chocolate (200 calories).

LUNCH: BBQ Pork Wrap
   8" whole-wheat tortilla wrap
   1 tsp onion powder
   2 tsp BBQ sauce
   2 tomato slices
   4 lettuce leaves
   6 oz pork loin

MID-AFTERNOON SNACK: Same as mid-morning snack.

DINNER: Lemon Baked Chicken, with rice and vegetable.

Family size (serves 4)	Single serving
Olive oil cooking spray	Olive oil cooking spray
2 tbsp fresh lemon juice	2 tsp fresh lemon juice
2 tbsp canola oil	2 tsp canola oil
1 clove of garlic, crushed	1/4 clove of garlic, crushed
1/2 tsp fresh ground pepper	fresh ground pepper to taste
2 1/2 lbs boneless, sk inless chicken breasts	8 oz boneless, skinless chicken breast

Preheat oven to 350 degrees. Lightly spray a baking pan or a shallow casserole dish with cooking spray. In a small bowl, combine lemon juice, oil, garlic and pepper. Set aside. Rinse chicken and pat dry. Arrange chicken in prepared pan or dish. Pour lemon mixture over chicken pieces. Cover and bake for 40 minutes, or until tender, basting occasionally. Uncover and bake 10 minutes longer to allow chicken to brown.

Serve with 6 oz (3/4 cup) of cooked brown or wild rice and 1 cup of any of the following steamed vegetables asparagus, broccoli, eggplant, green beans, kale, snow pea pods, or spinach.

1600 CALORIES

Week 3 * Day 6

BREAKFAST: One cup of cereal (see cereal choices) and one cup soy milk or low-fat or skim milk.

MID-MORNING SNACK: Snacks may consist of two of the following choices: banana; apple; pear; 2 cups strawberries (no sugar added); 1.5 cups blueberries (no sugar added); 2 cups raspberries (no sugar added); low-calorie yogurt (100 calories); 1 oz of soy nuts (100 calories total, varies based on brand and preparation); 1 oz soy chips (I recommend Revival brand soy chips. Three to four times a week, if desired, you may substitute any 200-calorie food you desire, for example two part-skim mozzarella cheese sticks or 2 oz of chocolate (200 calories).

LUNCH: Island Wrap
  8" whole-wheat tortilla wrap
  2 lettuce leaves
  6 oz ham
  3 slices tomato
  1 tsp bacon bits
  1 oz mozzarella cheese
  1 oz pineapple
  2 tsp fat-free ranch dressing

MID-AFTERNOON SNACK: Same as mid-morning snack.

DINNER: Spinach **Stuffed** Sirloin

Family size (serves 4)	Single serving
2 lb lean sirloin steak, 1" to 1 1/2" thick	8 oz lean sirloin steak, 1" to 1 1/2" thick
1- 10 oz pkg frozen spinach, thawed and drained	4 oz pkg frozen spinach, thawed and drained
2 cloves garlic, crushed	1/2 clove garlic, crushed
cooking oil spray	cooking oil spray
1/4 lb mushrooms, finely chopped	2 oz mushrooms, finely chopped
1/2 cup diced red bell pepper (optional)	2 oz diced red bell pepper (optional)
1 tbsp olive oil	1 tsp olive oil
1/4 cup grated parmesan cheese	1 oz grated Parmesan cheese

Preheat broiler. Meanwhile, heat oil in small sauté pan until hot but not smoking. Cook garlic, mushroom, and red bell pepper until softened. Add spinach and heat through. Stir in grated Parmesan thoroughly and remove from heat. With a sharp knife, cut pocket in sirloin steak nearly to the edges. Stuff with warm spinach mixture and place on rack in shallow pan. For medium rare, broil for 5 minutes on first side and 3 minutes, approximately, after turning steak over. For other doneness, adjust broiling time accordingly.

Serve with 6oz (3/4cup) of cooked brown or wild rice and 1 cup of any of the following steamed vegetables asparagus, broccoli, eggplant, green beans, kale, snow pea pods, or spinach.

1600 CALORIES

Week 3 * Day 7

BREAKFAST: One cup of cereal (see cereal choices) and one cup soy milk or low-fat or skim milk.

MID-MORNING SNACK: Snacks may consist of two of the following choices: banana; apple; pear; 2 cups strawberries (no sugar added); 1.5 cups blueberries (no sugar added); 2 cups raspberries (no sugar added); low-calorie yogurt (100 calories); 1 oz of soy nuts (100 calories total, varies based on brand and preparation); 1 oz soy chips (I recommend Revival brand soy chips. Three to four times a week, if desired, you may substitute any 200-calorie food you desire, for example two part-skim mozzarella cheese sticks or 2 oz of chocolate (200 calories).

LUNCH: BBQ Pork Burrito

8" whole-wheat tortilla wrap
3 lettuce leaves
2 oz chicken
3 tomato slices
1 oz corn

1 oz low-fat mozzarella cheese
3 oz black beans
1 tsp barbeque sauce
1 tsp sour cream

MID-AFTERNOON SNACK: Same as mid-morning snack.

DINNER: Chicken Manicotti, with rice and vegetable.

Family size (serves 4)
3/4 tsp oregano
1/2 tsp marjoram
3/4 tsp sweet basil
1/4 tsp fresh ground pepper
1- 6 oz can no-salt-added tomato paste
1 cup water
1 clove garlic, minced
4 boneless, skinless chicken breasts, (about 1 lb), fat removed
4 oz low-fat cottage cheese, drained
2 oz grated, part-skim mozzarella cheese

Single serving
1/4 tsp oregano
1 pinch marjoram
1/4 tsp sweet basil
1 pinch fresh ground pepper
2 oz can no-salt-added tomato paste
2 oz water
1/4 clove garlic, minced
1 boneless, skinless chicken breast, (6 oz), fat removed
1 oz low-fat cottage cheese, drained
1 oz grated, part-skim mozzarella

Preheat oven to 350 degrees. In a small bowl, combine first four spices. Mix well. Set aside. In a small saucepan, blend tomato paste, water, and garlic. Add 3/4 of the seasoning mixture to the pan. Bring to a boil. Reduce heat and simmer 10 minutes, stirring occasionally. Meanwhile, rinse chicken and pat dry. Place breast fillets in a plastic bag and pound to 1/4" thickness. Set aside in a small bowl, combine remaining spice mixture with cottage cheese. Spoon mixtures onto centers of chicken breasts, leaving a 1/2 inch edge all around. From narrow end, roll each breast, leaving a 1/2 inch edge all around. Spoon half of the tomato mixture into the bottom of a 10 x 6 inch baking dish. Arrange chicken roll on top, seam side down. Spoon remaining tomato mixture over the chicken rolls. Top with Mozzarella cheese and bake about 45 minutes, or until golden brown.

Serve with 6 oz (3/4 cup) of cooked brown or wild rice and 1 cup of any of the following steamed vegetables: asparagus, broccoli, eggplant, green beans, kale, snow pea pods, or spinach.

1800 CALORIE DIET

Calorie Distribution in 1800 Calorie Diet

Breakfast	350 Calories
Mid-Morning Snack	200 Calories
Lunch	475 Calories
Mid-Afternoon Snack	200 Calories
Dinner	575 Calories

Rules for the North Star Diet

1) Eat breakfast within 20 minutes after waking in the morning. Failure to eat a timely breakfast will decrease your fat-burning capacity, or metabolism. Breakfast choices consist of any high-fiber cereal with non-fat milk fortified with vitamin D and calcium or, preferably, non-fat soy milk fortified with vitamin D and calcium. High-fiber cereals should contain at least 8 grams of fiber in each serving. Recommended high-fiber cereals:

CEREAL	PORTION	CALORIES	FIBER (content)
General Mills Fiber One	1/2 cup	59	14 g
General Mills Fiber One Honey Clusters**	1 1/4 cup	170	14 g
Kellogg's Bran Buds	1/3 cup	80	11 g
Kellogg's All-Bran	1/2 cup	80	10 g
Post or Nabisco			
100% Bran	1/3 cup	80	9 g
Post Raisin Bran	1 cup	190	8 g
Kashi Good Friends	3/4 cup	90	8 g
Kashi Lean Crunch	1 cup	190	8 g
OATMEAL			
Quaker Weight Control	1 serving	160	8 g
TORTILLAS			
Cruz whole-wheat	large 8"	130	11 g
La tortilla factory	large 8"	80	14 g
Mission low carb	6" size	110	11 g

2) Consume mid-morning snacks and mid-afternoon snacks. Both snacks may consist of one (1200 calorie diet) or two (all other diets) of the following choices: banana; apple; pear; 2 cups strawberries (no sugar added); 1.5 cups blueberries (no sugar added); 2 cups raspberries (no sugar added); low-calorie yogurt (100 calories); 1 oz of soy nuts (100 calories total, varies based on brand and preparation); 1 oz soy chips (I recommend Revival brand soy chips). Failure to eat timely mid-morning and mid-afternoon snacks will decrease your fat-burning capacity, or metabolism. Three to four times a week you may substitute any food you desire(100 to 200 calories depending upon meal plan), for example one or two part-skim mozzarella cheese stick(s) or 1-2 oz of chocolate (100-200 calories).

Rules for the North Star Diet, cont'd.

3) Consume 2 liters of fluid a day (approximately 80 ounces). Eighty ounces of fluid is the equivalent of 8 ounces of water per hour for ten hours a day, or two 8-ounce glasses of water with each meal and snack. You may substitute diet soda pop or tea with meals if desired but no fruit juice or regular pop is allowed.

4) Consumption of two cups of green tea, one tea bag per cup, will promote 70 calories of weight loss on a daily basis. A personal favorite is Tazo Zen brand of green tea.

5) Consume dinner 3-4 hours prior to bedtime. If you eat closer to bedtime there is an increased chance the food will be stored and converted into fat while you sleep. If you are still hungry after dinner, you may consume an apple, pear or banana or 1 ounce of lean, grilled protein, e.g. turkey, ham, beef, or fish.

6) The meal plans are to be used as guides. Most individuals only eat 7-10 different foods in a given week. If yo u like certain wraps or dinners and not others, consume those you enjoy the most. I only ask that starting in the second week of the North Star Diet you begin utilizing a whole-wheat wrap/tortilla. (See lunch alternative if you desire to use bread as an alternative). Whole-wheat wraps can often contain as much as 10 –14 g of fiber per serving. They are easy to make. Combine fillings in the center of the tortilla and roll up. I recommend the following whole-wheat tortilla/wraps: Cruz brand whole-wheat tortilla (10 grams of dietary fiber per serving); La Tortilla Factory whol e-wheat, low-carb/low-fat tortillas (large size, 14 grams of fiber); and Carb Down flat bread (14 grams of fiber).

7) Consume daily: a multi-vitamin; 1200 mg of calcium carbonate; 1000 I.U. vitamin D; and 1000-3000 mg of fish oil.

** Personal Favorite

Measurement Conversions

Do not fear the measurements in the following calorie-specific diets. You could weigh each item as described. However, I approximate all food quantities based on the volume of a deck of playing cards.

3 ounces (oz) = the fluid volume of a deck of playing cards.

1 cup = 8 fluid ounces = 2.5 fluid equivalents of a deck of playing cards.

1 ounce (oz) = the fluid equivalent of one-third of a deck of playing cards.

1/2 ounce (oz) = 1 tablespoon (tbsp) = the fluid equivalent of 1/6 of a deck of playing cards.

1800 CALORIES

Week 1 * Day 1

BREAKFAST: One cup of cereal (see cereal choices) and one cup soy milk or low-fat or skim milk, and one of the following: banana; apple; pear; 2 cups of strawberries (no sugar added); 1.5 cups of blueberries (no sugar added); 2 cups of raspberries (no sugar added); or low-calorie yogurt (100 calories).

MID-MORNING SNACK: Snacks may consist of two of the following choices: banana; apple; pear; 2 cups strawberries (no sugar added); 1.5 cups blueberries (no sugar added); 2 cups raspberries (no sugar added); low-calorie yogurt (100 calories); 1 oz of soy nuts (100 calories total, varies based on brand and preparation); 1 oz soy chips (I recommend Revival brand soy chips. Three to four times a week, if desired, you may substitute any 200-calorie food you desire, for example two part-skim mozzarella cheese sticks or 2 oz of chocolate (200 calories).

LUNCH: Mediterranean Wrap
  8" tortilla wrap
  6 oz turkey, roasted or sliced, skinless white meat
  4 lettuce leaves
  2 oz cucumber strips
  1 tsp red pepper flakes
  1 oz feta cheese
  2 tsp fat-free red wine vinegar

MID-AFTERNOON SNACK: Same as mid-morning snack.

DINNER: Crispy Baked Chicken, with rice and vegetable.

Family size (4 servings)	Single serving
3 lbs boneless, skinless chicken breasts	10 oz boneless, skinless chicken breast
1 cup skim milk	1/4 cup skim milk
1 cup cornflake crumbs	1/4 cup cornflake crumbs
1 tsp rosemary	1 pinch rosemary
1 tsp fresh ground black pepper	1 pinch fresh ground black pepper
Pam cooking oil spray or olive oil spray	Pam cooking oil spray or olive oil spray

Preheat oven to 350 degrees. Cover a baking dish with foil and spray lightly with cooking oil spray. Rinse chicken and pat dry. Set aside. Pour milk into a shallow bowl. Combine cornflake crumbs, rosemary, and pepper in another shallow bowl. Dip chicken into milk and then into crumb mixture. Allow to stand briefly so coating will adhere. Arrange chicken in prepared pan so pieces do not touch. Bake 40 minutes or until done. Crumbs will form a crisp "skin".

Serve with 3/4 cup of cooked wild or brown rice and 1 cup of any of the following vegetables: asparagus, broccoli, eggplant, green beans, kale, snow pea pod pods or spinach.

1800 CALORIES

Week 1 * Day 2

BREAKFAST: One cup of cereal (see cereal choices) and one cup soy milk or low-fat or skim milk, and one of the following: banana; apple; pear; 2 cups of strawberries (no sugar added); 1.5 cups of blueberries (no sugar added); 2 cups of raspberries (no sugar added); or low-calorie yogurt (100 calories).

MID-MORNING SNACK: Snacks may consist of two of the following choices: banana; apple; pear; 2 cups strawberries (no sugar added); 1.5 cups blueberries (no sugar added); 2 cups raspberries (no sugar added); low-calorie yogurt (100 calories); 1 oz of soy nuts (100 calories total, varies based on brand and preparation); 1 oz soy chips (I recommend Revival brand soy chips. Three to four times a week, if desired, you may substitute any 200-calorie food you desire, for example two part-skim mozzarella cheese sticks or 2 oz of chocolate (200 calories).

LUNCH: Beef Taquito Wrap
  8" tortilla wrap
  4 oz round steak, trimmed
  1 oz mozzarella low-fat cheese
  2 tsp salsa

MID-AFTERNOON SNACK: Same as mid-morning snack.

DINNER: Scallops Oriental, with rice and vegetable.

Family size (4 servings)
  cooking oil spray (preferably olive oil)
  2 lb fresh or frozen scallops
  1/8 cup honey
  1/8 cup mustard
  1/2 tsp curry powder
  1/2 tsp lemon juice

Single serving
  cooking oil spray (preferably olive oil)
  8 oz of fresh or frozen scallops
  2 tsp of honey
  2 tsp mustard
  pinch curry powder
  1/8 tsp lemon juice

Preheat broiler. Lightly spray baking pan with cooking spray. Rinse scallops and drain. Place in a baking pan. In a saucepan, combine remaining ingredients. Brush scallops with sauce. Broil 4 inches from heat for 5-8 minutes or until browned.

Serve with 3/4 cup of cooked wild or brown rice and 1 cup of any of the following steamed vegetables: asparagus, broccoli, eggplant, green beans, kale, snow pea pods, or spinach.

1800 CALORIES

Week 1 * Day 3

BREAKFAST: One cup of cereal (see cereal choices) and one cup soy milk or low-fat or skim milk, and one of the following: banana; apple; pear; 2 cups of strawberries (no sugar added); 1.5 cups of blueberries (no sugar added); 2 cups of raspberries (no sugar added); or low-calorie yogurt (100 calories).

MID-MORNING SNACK: Snacks may consist of two of the following choices: banana; apple; pear; 2 cups strawberries (no sugar added); 1.5 cups blueberries (no sugar added); 2 cups raspberries (no sugar added); low-calorie yogurt (100 calories); 1 oz of soy nuts (100 calories total, varies based on brand and preparation); 1 oz soy chips (I recommend Revival brand soy chips. Three to four times a week, if desired, you may substitute any 200-calorie food you desire, for example two part-skim mozzarella cheese sticks or 2 oz of chocolate (200 calories).

Lunch: Tuna Mayo Wrap
   8" tortilla wrap
   2 oz low-fat mayonnaise
   8 oz tuna
   1/4 rib celery

MID-AFTERNOON SNACK: Same as mid-morning snack.

DINNER: Tomato, Mushroom, and Jack Cheese Omelet, with vegetable and baked potato.

Single Serving
   Cooking oil spray (olive oil preferable)
   4 eggs or egg substitute equivalent
   1/4 cup seeded, chopped tomato
   1/2 oz shredded, low-fat Monterey jack cheese
   1/4 cup mushrooms
   1 tsp chopped cilantro or parsley
   Hot pepper sauce (optional)

Spray skillet with cooking oil, or use non-stick frying pan. Place pan over medium-high heat. In a small bowl, place eggs or egg substitute . Beat and pour mixture into pan. Stir eggs in a circular motion. Do not scrape bottom of pan. When the omelet is almost cooked, add fillings. Fold omelet over with a fork while holding the pan at 45-degree angle. Roll omelet onto plate and serve.

Serve with 1 large (8-9 oz) baked potato with 1 tsp soft canola margarine, and 1 cup of any of the following steamed vegetables: asparagus, broccoli, eggplant, green beans, kale, snow pea pods, or spinach.

1800 CALORIES

Week 1 * Day 4

BREAKFAST: One cup of cereal (see cereal choices) and one cup soy milk or low-fat or skim milk, and one of the following: banana; apple; pear; 2 cups of strawberries (no sugar added); 1.5 cups of blueberries (no sugar added); 2 cups of raspberries (no sugar added); or low-calorie yogurt (100 calories).

MID-MORNING SNACK: Snacks may consist of two of the following choices: banana; apple; pear; 2 cups strawberries (no sugar added); 1.5 cups blueberries (no sugar added); 2 cups raspberries (no sugar added); low-calorie yogurt (100 calories); 1 oz of soy nuts (100 calories total, varies based on brand and preparation); 1 oz soy chips (I recommend Revival brand soy chips. Three to four times a week, if desired, you may substitute any 200-calorie food you desire, for example two part-skim mozzarella cheese sticks or 2 oz of chocolate (200 calories).

LUNCH: Beef Wrap
   8" whole-wheat tortilla wrap
   6 oz broiled, trimmed round steak
   1/2 cup raw or broiled mushrooms
   2 tsp Worcestershire sauce
   1 tsp soy sauce

MID-AFTERNOON SNACK: Same as mid-morning snack.

DINNER: Mustard-Crusted Pork, with rice and vegetable.

Serving for two
   2 tsp soy or tofu flour (available at most health food stores)
   1 tsp mustard powder
   1/2 tsp pepper
   1/4 cup olive oil
   1 1/2 lb boneless, center-cut pork chops, cut against the grain into 3" strips, about 3/8 " thick

Single serving
   2 tsp soy or tofu flour (available at most health food stores)
   1 tsp mustard powder
   1/2 tsp pepper
   1/4 cup olive oil
   12 oz boneless, center-cut pork chops, cut against the grain into 3" strips, about 3/8 " thick

Combine the flour, mustard powder, and pepper in a bowl and mix well. Dust the pork with the flour mixture. Heat 2 tbs oil over medium heat until hot but not smoking. Add half the pork and brown for five minutes on each side, or until cooked through. Repeat with the remaining pork. Sprinkle with seasoning. Remove from he at and serve immediately.

Serve with 3/4 cup of cooked wild or brown rice and 1 cup of any of the following steamed vegetables: asparagus, broccoli, eggplant, green beans, kale, snow pea pods, or spinach.

1800 CALORIES

Week 1 * Day 5

BREAKFAST: One cup of cereal (see cereal choices) and one cup soy milk or low-fat or skim milk, and one of the following: banana; apple; pear; 2 cups of strawberries (no sugar added); 1.5 cups of blueberries (no sugar added); 2 cups of raspberries (no sugar added); or low-calorie yogurt (100 calories).

MID-MORNING SNACK: Snacks may consist of two of the following choices: banana; apple; pear; 2 cups strawberries (no sugar added); 1.5 cups blueberries (no sugar added); 2 cups raspberries (no sugar added); low-calorie yogurt (100 calories); 1 oz of soy nuts (100 calories total, varies based on brand and preparation); 1 oz soy chips (I recommend Revival brand soy chips. Three to four times a week, if desired, you may substitute any 200-scalorie food you desire, for example two part-skim mozzarella cheese sticks or 2 oz of chocolate (200 calories).

LUNCH: Turkey Vegetable Wraps
   8" tortilla wrap
   6 oz turkey, roasted or sliced, skinless white meat
   1 oz corn, canned in water
   1 oz red pepper
   1 oz green onion
   2 tsp fat-free, light ranch dressing

MID-AFTERNOON SNACK: Same as mid-morning snack.

DINNER: Fish Fillets with Asparagus, with rice and vegetable.

Family size (serves four)	Single serving
Cooking oil spray (preferably olive oil)	Cooking oil spray (preferably olive oil)
4 - 9 oz mild, white fish fillets (Haddock, cod, etc.)	1 - 9 oz mild, white fish fillet
1/2 tsp ground black pepper	(Haddock, cod, etc.)
2 tbsp unsalted butter	1/4 tsp ground black pepper
12 stalks cooked asparagus	1 tbsp unsalted butter
1/3 cup tangy sour cream	3 stalks cooked asparagus
1/3 cup plain low-fat yogurt	1/3 cup tangy sour cream
2 tsp minced chives	1/3 cup plain low-fat yogurt
2 tsp horseradish	1 tsp minced chives
1 egg white	1 tsp horseradish
2 tsp chopped parsley	1 egg white
	1 tsp chopped parsley

Preheat broiler. Lightly spray broiler pan with cooking spray. Rinse fish and pat dry. Season fish with pepper and lemon juice and brush with margarine. Place on broiler pan and broil about 8 minutes or until fish almost flakes. Remove from oven and top each fillet with 3 stalks of asparagus. In a small bowl, combine sour cream, yogurt, chives, horseradish, and dill weed. In another bowl, beat egg whites until stiff peaks form; fold into sour cream mixture. Spread mixture over each fillet to cover fish and asparagus. Return to broiler and broil 1-2 minutes, or until golden brown. Sprinkle with parsley.

Serve with 3/4 cup of cooked wild or brown rice and 1 cup of any of the following vegetables: asparagus, broccoli, eggplant, green beans, kale, snow pea pod pods or spinach.

1800 CALORIES

Week 1 * Day 6

BREAKFAST: One cup of cereal (see cereal choices) and one cup soy milk or low-fat or skim milk, and one of the following: banana; apple; pear; 2 cups of strawberries (no sugar added); 1.5 cups of blueberries (no sugar added); 2 cups of raspberries (no sugar added); or low-calorie yogurt (100 calories).

MID-MORNING SNACK: Snacks may consist of two of the following choices: banana; apple; pear; 2 cups strawberries (no sugar added); 1.5 cups blueberries (no sugar added); 2 cups raspberries (no sugar added); low-calorie yogurt (100 calories); 1 oz of soy nuts (100 calories total, varies based on brand and preparation); 1 oz soy chips (I recommend Revival brand soy chips. Three to four times a week, if desired, you may substitute any 200-calorie food you desire, for example two part-skim mozzarella cheese sticks or 2 oz of chocolate (200 calories).

LUNCH: California Chicken Wrap
   8" whole-wheat tortilla wrap
   5 oz grilled white chicken
   2 tsp guacamole
   3 slices tomato
   3 lettuce leaves
   1 tsp bacon bits

MID-AFTERNOON SNACK: Same as mid-morning snack.

DINNER: Feta Burgers, with rice and steamed vegetable.

Family size (serves 4)	Single serving
cooking oil spray, preferably olive oil	8 oz ground sirloin or ground round
2 lb ground sirloin or ground round	1 oz feta cheese
1/4 cup crumbled feta cheese	1 oz finely chopped black olives
1/4 cup finely chopped black olives	1/2 tsp salt
1/2 tsp salt	1/2 tsp pepper
1/2 tsp pepper	

Heat pan sprayed with cooking spray. Mix remaining ingredients and shape into four patties (one for single serving). Sauté patties at medium high heat for 5 minutes on each side or to desired doneness.

Serve with 3/4 cup of cooked wild or brown rice and 1 cup of any of the following steamed vegetables: asparagus, broccoli, eggplant, green beans, kale, snow pea pods, or spinach.

1800 CALORIES

Week 1 * Day 7

BREAKFAST: One cup of cereal (see cereal choices) and one cup soy milk or low-fat or skim milk, and one of the following: banana; apple; pear; 2 cups of strawberries (no sugar added); 1.5 cups of blueberries (no sugar added); 2 cups of raspberries (no sugar added); or low-calorie yogurt (100 calories).

MID-MORNING SNACK: Snacks may consist of two of the following choices: banana; apple; pear; 2 cups strawberries (no sugar added); 1.5 cups blueberries (no sugar added); 2 cups raspberries (no sugar added); low-calorie yogurt (100 calories); 1 oz of soy nuts (100 calories total, varies based on brand and preparation); 1 oz soy chips (I recommend Revival brand soy chips. Three to four times a week, if desired, you may substitute any 200-calorie food you desire, for example two part-skim mozzarella cheese sticks or 2 oz of chocolate (200 calories).

LUNCH: Ham Club Wrap
   8" whole-wheat tortilla wrap
   6 oz ham
   3 slices tomato
   3 lettuce leaves
   1 tsp bacon bits
   1 tsp light Italian dressing
   1 oz low-fat mozzarella cheese

MID-AFTERNOON SNACK: Same as mid-morning snack.

DINNER: Lemon Baked Chicken, with rice and steamed vegetable.

Family size (serves 4)	Single serving
olive oil cooking spray	olive oil cooking spray
2 tsp fresh lemon juice	1 tsp fresh lemon juice
2 tsp low-fat margarine or safflower oil	1 tsp low-fat margarine or safflower oil
1 clove garlic, crushed	1/4 clove garlic, crushed
1/2 tsp fresh ground black pepper	1/8 tsp fresh ground black pepper
2 lbs boneless, skinless chicken breast.	10 oz boneless, skinless chicken breast

Preheat oven to 350 degrees. Lightly spray a baking pan or a shallow casserole dish with cooking spray. In a small bowl, combine lemon juice, oil, garlic and pepper. Set aside. Rinse chicken and pat dry. Arrange chicken in prepared pan or dish. Pour lemon mixture over chicken pieces. Cover and bake 40 minutes or until tender, basting occasionally. Uncover and bake 10 minutes longer to allow chicken to brown.

Serve with 3/4 cup of cooked wild or brown rice and 1 cup of any of the following steamed vegetables: asparagus, broccoli, eggplant, green beans, kale, snow pea pods, or spinach.

1800 CALORIES

Week 2 * Day 1

BREAKFAST: One cup of cereal (see cereal choices) and one cup soy milk or low-fat or skim milk, and one of the following: banana; apple; pear; 2 cups of strawberries (no sugar added); 1.5 cups of blueberries (no sugar added); 2 cups of raspberries (no sugar added); or low-calorie yogurt (100 calories).

MID-MORNING SNACK: Snacks may consist of two of the following choices: banana; apple; pear; 2 cups strawberries (no sugar added); 1.5 cups blueberries (no sugar added); 2 cups raspberries (no sugar added); low-calorie yogurt (100 calories); 1 oz of soy nuts (100 calories total, varies based on brand and preparation); 1 oz soy chips (I recommend Revival brand soy chips. Threet of our times a week, if desired, you may substitute any 200-calorie food you desire, for example two part-skim mozzarella cheese sticks or 2 oz of chocolate (200 calories).

LUNCH: Chicken with Zucchini and Roasted Pepper Wrap
    8" whole-wheat tortilla wrap
    6 oz broiled white chicken meat
    3-4 oz zucchini
    2 oz pickled sweet peppers
    1 oz part-skim, reduced-fat mozzarella cheese

MID-AFTERNOON SNACK: Same as mid-morning snack.

DINNER: Pineapple and Shrimp, with rice and vegetable

Family size (Serves 4)	Single serving
1 clove garlic, crushed	1 tsp garlic powder or 1/4 clove garlic, crushed
2 tbsp canola margarine	2 tsp canola margarine
1/4 cup honey	1 oz honey
1 tbsp sweet chili sauce	1 tsp sweet chili sauce
1 tbsp soy sauce	1 tsp of soy sauce
1 whole pineapple, or 20 oz canned in water or light syrup	6 oz fresh pineapple, or 6 oz canned in water or light syrup
2 1/2 lbs of shrimp, fresh or frozen, peeled and de-veined	10 oz shrimp, fresh or frozen, peeled and de-veined

Combine first five ingredients in a bowl. Brush shrimp with the mixture. Grill at high temperature for 5 minutes. Add pineapple.

Serve with 3/4 cup of cooked wild or brown rice and 1 cup of any of the following steamed vegetables: asparagus, broccoli, eggplant, green beans, kale, snow pea pods, or spinach.

1800 CALORIES

Week 2 * Day 2

BREAKFAST: One cup of cereal (see cereal choices) and one cup soy milk or low-fat or skim milk, and one of the following: banana; apple; pear; 2 cups of strawberries (no sugar added); 1.5 cups of blueberries (no sugar added); 2 cups of raspberries (no sugar added); or low-calorie yogurt (100 calories).

MID-MORNING SNACK: Snacks may consist of two of the following choices: banana; apple; pear; 2 cups strawberries (no sugar added); 1.5 cups blueberries (no sugar added); 2 cups raspberries (no sugar added); low-calorie yogurt (100 calories); 1 oz of soy nuts (100 calories total, varies based on brand and preparation); 1 oz soy chips (I recommend Revival brand soy chips. Three to four times a week, if desired, you may substitute any 200-calorie food you desire, for example two part-skim mozzarella cheese sticks or 2 oz of chocolate (200 calories).

LUNCH: Santa Fe Steak Burrito
   8" whole-wheat tortilla wrap
   2 oz steak
   1 oz corn
   3 oz black beans
   1 tsp sour cream
   3 lettuce leaves
   3 tomato slices
   1 oz low-fat mozzarella cheese
   2 tsp salsa

MID-AFTERNOON SNACK: Same as mid-morning snack.

DINNER: Turkey Burgers, with wild rice and vegetable.

Family size (serves 4)	Single serving
2 lb ground turkey (90% lean), thawed	8 oz ground turkey (90% lean), thawed
1/4 cup onions, or powdered onion flakes	1 oz onions, or powdered onion flakes
2 tbsp green peppers	2 tsp green peppers
1 tbsp Worcestershire sauce	1 tsp Worcestershire sauce
2 tbsp ketchup	1 tsp ketchup
1/4 tsp black pepper	1/8 tsp black pepper
lettuce leaves	lettuce leaves
tomato slices	tomato slices
4 whole-wheat pita pockets	1 whole-wheat pita pocket

Form ground turkey and seasoning into patties. Grill or broil for 5 minutes per side, or until done. Top patties with lettuce and tomato and place in pita pocket.

Serve with 4 oz (1/2 cup) of cooked brown or wild rice and 1 cup of any of the following steamed vegetables: asparagus, broccoli, eggplant, green beans, kale, snow pea pods, or spinach.

1800 CALORIES

Week 2 *Day 3

BREAKFAST: One cup of cereal (see cereal choices) and one cup soy milk or low-fat or skim milk, and one of the following: banana; apple; pear; 2 cups of strawberries (no sugar added); 1.5 cups of blueberries (no sugar added); 2 cups of raspberries (no sugar added); or low-calorie yogurt (100 calories).

MID-MORNING SNACK: Snacks may consist of two of the following choices: banana; apple; pear; 2 cups strawberries (no sugar added); 1.5 cups blueberries (no sugar added); 2 cups raspberries (no sugar added); low-calorie yogurt (100 calories); 1 oz of soy nuts (100 calories total, varies based on brand and preparation); 1 oz soy chips (I recommend Revival brand soy chips. Three to four times a week, if desired, you may substitute any 200-calorie food you desire, for example two part-skim mozzarella cheese sticks or 2 oz of chocolate (200 calories).

LUNCH: Tasty Turkey Wrap
   8" whole-wheat tortilla wrap
   onion powder to taste
   6 oz turkey
   2 tsp sliced olives
   1 oz mozzarella low-fat cheese
   2 tsp fat-free mayo
   3 lettuce leaves
   1 tsp mustard
   3 slices tomato

MID-AFTERNOON SNACK: Same as mid-morning snack.

DINNER: Chicken with Mushrooms, with baked potato and vegetable.

Family size (serves 4)	Single serving
4 - 10 oz chicken breasts, skinless	1 - 10 oz chicken breast, skinless
20 oz button mushrooms	5 oz button mushrooms
1/2 tsp pepper	1/2 tsp pepper
2 tbsp olive oil	1 garlic clove
juice of half a lemon	1 tbsp olive oil
1 cup dry white wine	juice of 1/4 lemon
pinch of dried hot red pepper flakes	1/2 cup dry white wine
	pinch of dried hot red pepper flakes

Grill chicken, set aside. Heat oil in a heavy skillet over medium heat. Add the garlic, lemon juice, wine, pepper, and red pepper flakes. Bring to a boil. Lower heat and add mushrooms. Simmer and stir frequently for 5 –6 minutes. Add pre-grilled chicken.

Serve with 1 medium (7 oz) baked potato with 1 tsp soft canola margarine, and 1 cup of any of the following steamed vegetables: asparagus, broccoli, eggplant, green beans, kale, snow pea pods, or spinach.

1800 CALORIES

Week 2 * Day 4

BREAKFAST: One cup of cereal (see cereal choices) and one cup soy milk or low-fat or skim milk, and one of the following: banana; apple; pear; 2 cups of strawberries (no sugar added); 1.5 cups of blueberries (no sugar added); 2 cups of raspberries (no sugar added); or low-calorie yogurt (100 calories).

MID-MORNING SNACK: Snacks may consist of two of the following choices: banana; apple; pear; 2 cups strawberries (no sugar added); 1.5 cups blueberries (no sugar added); 2 cups raspberries (no sugar added); low-calorie yogurt (100 calories); 1 oz of soy nuts (100 calories total, varies based on brand and preparation); 1 oz soy chips (I recommend Revival brand soy chips. Three to four times a week, if desired, you may substitute any 200-calorie food you desire, for example two part-skim mozzarella cheese sticks or 2 oz of chocolate (200 calories).

LUNCH: Greek Wrap
   8" whole-wheat tortilla wrap
   6 oz grilled chicken breast, no skin
   1 oz feta cheese (reduced fat)
   4 lettuce leaves
   2-3 tomato slices
   2 tsp low-calorie vinaigrette dressing

MID-AFTERNOON SNACK: Same as mid-morning snack.

DINNER: Pork with Green Chile and Cheese, and rice and vegetable.

Family size (serves 4)
   2 1/2 lbs boneless, center-cut loin pork chops or sirloin pork steaks (fat removed)
   2 tbsp olive oil
   1/2 cup green chili salsa
   3/4 cup low-fat cheese, shredded (feta, Muenster, cheddar, or mozzarella)

Single serving
   10 oz boneless, center-cut loin pork chops or sirloin pork steaks (fat removed)
   1 tsp olive oil
   2 oz green chili salsa
   2 oz low-fat cheese, shredded (feta, Muenster, cheddar, or mozzarella)

Heat oil in pan over medium heat until hot but not smoking. Add pork to pan and brown for 3-5 minutes. Turn heat to low, add 1/2 cup water, and cover pan. Cook for 20-25 minutes or until water is nearly evaporated. Pour salsa over pork, covering evenly. Sprinkle with shredded cheese, cover and cook for additional 3 to 5 minutes or until salsa is heated and cheese is melted.

Serve immediately with 6 oz (3/4 cup) of cooked brown or wild rice and 1 cup of any of the following steamed vegetables: asparagus, broccoli, eggplant, green beans, kale, snow pea pods, or spinach.

1800 CALORIES

Week 2 * Day 5

BREAKFAST: One cup of cereal (see cereal choices) and one cup soy milk or low-fat or skim milk, and one of the following: banana; apple; pear; 2 cups of strawberries (no sugar added); 1.5 cups of blueberries (no sugar added); 2 cups of raspberries (no sugar added); or low-calorie yogurt (100 calories).

MID-MORNING SNACK: Snacks may consist of two of the following choices: banana; apple; pear; 2 cups strawberries (no sugar added); 1.5 cups blueberries (no sugar added); 2 cups raspberries (no sugar added); low-calorie yogurt (100 calories); 1 oz of soy nuts (100 calories total, varies based on brand and preparation); 1 oz soy chips (I recommend Revival brand soy chips. Three to four times a week, if desired, you may substitute any 200-calorie food you desire, for example two part-skim mozzarella cheese sticks or 2 oz of chocolate (200 calories).

LUNCH: Bean and Cheese Burrito
    8" whole-wheat tortilla wrap
    3 oz reduced-fat cheddar cheese
    7 oz black beans
    3 lettuce leaves

Heat, if desired, in microwave or toaster oven.

MID-AFTERNOON SNACK: Same as mid-morning snack.

DINNER: Tandoori Chicken, with rice and vegetable.

Family Size (serves 4)
    4 - 10 oz chicken breasts, skinless
    3 tsp tandoori spice mix
    1 tsp fresh ginger, grated
    1 1/2 cups plain, non-fat yogurt

Single serving
    1 - 10 oz chicken breast, skinless
    1 tsp tandoori spice mix
    1/3 tsp fresh ginger, grated
    1/2 cups plain, non-fat yogurt

Mix yogurt, tandoori spice, cumin and ginger in a bowl. Brush mixture on chicken breasts. Grill on high for 2 minutes on each side. Reduce heat and cook 5 minutes longer on each side, basting while cooking.

Serve with 6 oz (3/4 cup) of cooked brown or wild rice and 1 cup of any of the following steamed vegetables: asparagus, broccoli, eggplant, green beans, kale, snow pea pods, or spinach.

1800 CALORIES

Week 2 * Day 6

BREAKFAST: One cup of cereal (see cereal choices) and one cup soy milk or low-fat or skim milk, and one of the following: banana; apple; pear; 2 cups of strawberries (no sugar added); 1.5 cups of blueberries (no sugar added); 2 cups of raspberries (no sugar added); or low-calorie yogurt (100 calories).

MID-MORNING SNACK: Snacks may consist of two of the following choices: banana; apple; pear; 2 cups strawberries (no sugar added); 1.5 cups blueberries (no sugar added); 2 cups raspberries (no sugar added); low-calorie yogurt (100 calories); 1 oz of soy nuts (100 calories total, varies based on brand and preparation); 1 oz soy chips (I recommend Revival brand soy chips. Three to four times a week, if desired, you may substitute any 200-calorie food you desire, for example two part-skim mozzarella cheese sticks or 2 oz of chocolate (200 calories).

LUNCH: Chicken Taquito
   8" whole-wheat tortilla wrap
   1 oz low-fat cheddar cheese
   6 oz white chicken meat
   2 tsp salsa

Heat in microwave or in toaster oven

MID-AFTERNOON SNACK: Same as mid-morning snack.

DINNER: Shrimp Scampi, with rice and vegetable.

Family size (serves 4)	Single serving
4 tbsp butter (unsalted)	1 tbsp butter (unsalted)
4 tbsp olive oil	1 tbsp olive oil
6 large cloves garlic, minced	1-2 large cloves garlic minced
1/2 cup chopped, fresh **flat-leaf** parsley	2 oz or 1/8 cup chopped, fresh **flat-leaf** parsley
juice of 1 lemon	juice of 1/4 lemon
1 cup dry white wine	2 oz or 1/4 cup of dry white wine
2 pinches dried, hot red pepper **flak**es	1 pinch of dried, hot red pepper **flakes**
salt and black pepper to taste.	salt and black pepper to taste
3 lbs large shrimp, shelled and de-veined, frozen or fresh	12 oz large shrimp, shelled and de-veined, frozen or fresh

Heat the butter and oil in a skillet over medium heat until the foam subsides. Add the garlic, parsley, lemon juice, wine, pepper **flakes,** salt and pepper. Bring to a boil, lower the heat, and simmer for 3 minutes. Add the shrimp to the skillet and cook, stirring frequently, for 5 to 6 minutes until the shrimp are pink. Remove from heat. Place the shrimp on a serving plate and pour the sauce from the skillet over them.

Serve immediately with 6 oz (3/4cup) of cooked brown or wild rice and 1 cup of any of the following steamed vegetables: asparagus, broccoli, eggplant, green beans, kale, snow peapods, or spinach.

1800 CALORIES

Week 2 * Day 7

BREAKFAST: One cup of cereal (see cereal choices) and one cup soy milk or low-fat or skim milk, and one of the following: banana; apple; pear; 2 cups of strawberries (no sugar added); 1.5 cups of blueberries (no sugar added); 2 cups of raspberries (no sugar added); or low-calorie yogurt (100 calories).

MID-MORNING SNACK: Snacks may consist of two of the following choices: banana; apple; pear; 2 cups strawberries (no sugar added); 1.5 cups blueberries (no sugar added); 2 cups raspberries (no sugar added); low-calorie yogurt (100 calories); 1 oz of soy nuts (100 calories total, varies based on brand and preparation); 1 oz soy chips (I recommend Revival brand soy chips. Three to four times a week, if desired, you may substitute any 200-calorie food you desire, for example two part-skim mozzarella cheese sticks or 2 oz of chocolate (200 calories).

LUNCH: Vegetarian Greek Wrap
   8" whole-wheat tortilla wrap
   1 oz black olives
   2 tbsp guacamole
   2 oz cucumber
   3 slices of tomato
   1 oz feta cheese (reduced-fat)
   4 oz hummus

MID-AFTERNOON SNACK: Same as mid-morning snack.

DINNER: Grilled Spicy Chicken Breast Fillets, with rice and vegetable.

Family size (Serves 4)	Single serving
1 small clove garlic, crushed	1 small clove garlic, crushed
1 small onion, finely chopped	1 small onion, finely chopped
2-3 tbsp lime juice	2-3 tbsp lime juice
2 tbsp olive oil	2 tbsp olive oil
1/2 tsp chili powder	1/2 tsp chili powder
fresh ground pepper to taste	fresh ground pepper to taste
4 - 10 oz boneless, skinless chicken breasts	1 - 10 oz boneless, skinless chicken breast

In a small bowl, combine ingredients. Coat chicken pieces thoroughly. On preheated grill or in broiler, cook chicken, turning once, 6-7 minutes, or until done.

Serve with 6 oz (3/4 cup) of cooked brown or wild rice and 1 cup of any of the following steamed vegetables: asparagus, broccoli, eggplant, green beans, kale, snow pea pods, or spinach.

1800 CALORIES

Week 3 * Day 1

BREAKFAST: One cup of cereal (see cereal choices) and one cup soy milk or low-fat or skim milk, and one of the following: banana; apple; pear; 2 cups of strawberries (no sugar added); 1.5 cups of blueberries (no sugar added); 2 cups of raspberries (no sugar added); or low-calorie yogurt (100 calories).

MID-MORNING SNACK: Snacks may consist of two of the following choices: banana; apple; pear; 2 cups strawberries (no sugar added); 1.5 cups blueberries (no sugar added); 2 cups raspberries (no sugar added); low-calorie yogurt (100 calories); 1 oz of soy nuts (100 calories total, varies based on brand and preparation); 1 oz soy chips (I recommend Revival brand soy chips. Three to four times a week, if desired, you may substitute any 200-calorie food you desire, for example two part-skim mozzarella cheese sticks or 2 oz of chocolate (200 calories).

LUNCH: Ham and Cheese Wrap
  8" whole-wheat tortilla wrap
  6 oz Healthy Choice ham (low-fat ham)
  2 tsp mustard
  1 oz cheddar cheese (low-fat if available)

MID-AFTERNOON SNACK: Same as mid-morning snack.

DINNER: Caribbean Grilled Tuna, with rice and vegetable.

Family size (serves 4)
  cooking oil spray
  4 – 10 oz tuna steaks
  1 tbsp lime and lemon juice
  3 tbsp olive oil
  1 tbsp of Caribbean Jerk Seasoning or Old Bay crab spice mixture

Single serving
  cooking oil spray
  1 - 10 oz tuna steak
  1 tsp lime and lemon juice
  1 tbsp olive oil
  1 tsp Caribbean Jerk Seasoning or Old Bay crab spice mixture

Mix together juice, oil, and seasonings. Brush mixture on to tuna steaks. Spray pan with olive oil cooking spray. Preheat grill or broiler pan. Place tuna on broiler. Grill or broil 5 minutes per side or until fish flakes with a fork.

Serve with 1 cup of cooked brown or wild rice and 1 cup of any of the following steamed vegetables: asparagus, broccoli, eggplant, green beans, kale, snow pea pods, or spinach.

1800 CALORIES

Week 3 * Day 2

BREAKFAST: One cup of cereal (see cereal choices) and one cup soy milk or low-fat or skim milk, and one of the following: banana; apple; pear; 2 cups of strawberries (no sugar added); 1.5 cups of blueberries (no sugar added); 2 cups of raspberries (no sugar added); or low-calorie yogurt (100 calories).

MID-MORNING SNACK: Snacks may consist of two of the following choices: banana; apple; pear; 2 cups strawberries (no sugar added); 1.5 cups blueberries (no sugar added); 2 cups raspberries (no sugar added); low-calorie yogurt (100 calories); 1 oz of soy nuts (100 calories total, varies based on brand and preparation); 1 oz soy chips (I recommend Revival brand soy chips. Three to four times a week, if desired, you may substitute any 200-calorie food you desire, for example two part-skim mozzarella cheese sticks or 2 oz of chocolate (200 calories).

LUNCH: Bar-B-Q Chicken Quesadilla
    8" whole-wheat tortilla wrap
    5 oz chicken
    2 tsp BBQ sauce
    1 1/2 oz reduced-fat cheddar cheese

MID-AFTERNOON SNACK: Same as mid-morning snack.

DINNER: Lemon Pepper Beef Steak, with baked potato and vegetable.

Family size (serves 4)
    2 1/4 lbs of lean beef steak, sirloin tip or round
    1 tsp olive oil
    2 garlic cloves, crushed
    2 tsp oregano
    1/2 tsp lemon pepper salt

Single serving
    9 oz lean beef steak, sirloin tip or round
    1 tsp olive oil
    1 garlic clove, crushed
    1 tsp oregano
    1/4 tsp lemon pepper salt

Combine seasoning ingredients in a bowl. Brush seasonings on steak. Broil steak until desired doneness.

Serve with 1 small (6 oz) baked potato with 1 tsp soft canola margarine, and 1 cup of any of the following steamed vegetables: asparagus, broccoli, eggplant, green beans, kale, snow pea pods, or spinach.

1800 CALORIES

Week 3 * Day 3

BREAKFAST: One cup of cereal (see cereal choices) and one cup soy milk or low-fat or skim milk, and one of the following: banana; apple; pear; 2 cups of strawberries (no sugar added); 1.5 cups of blueberries (no sugar added); 2 cups of raspberries (no sugar added); or low-calorie yogurt (100 calories).

MID-MORNING SNACK: Snacks may consist of two of the following choices: banana; apple; pear; 2 cups strawberries (no sugar added); 1.5 cups blueberries (no sugar added); 2 cups raspberries (no sugar added); low-calorie yogurt (100 calories); 1 oz of soy nuts (100 calories total, varies based on brand and preparation); 1 oz soy chips (I recommend Revival brand soy chips. Three to four times a week, if desired, you may substitute any 200-calorie food you desire, for example two part-skim mozzarella cheese sticks or 2 oz of chocolate (200 calories).

LUNCH: Garlic Chicken Burrito
  8" whole-wheat tortilla wrap
  3 lettuce leaves
  4 oz chicken
  1 slice tomato
  1 tsp garlic powder
  1 tsp sour cream
  1 oz corn
  1 oz low-fat mozzarella cheese
  3 oz black beans

MID-AFTERNOON SNACK: Same as mid-morning snack.

DINNER: 2 Crab Cakes, with vegetable.

Family size (serves 4)
  1 egg beaten
  2 slices bread, crust removed, broken into crumbs
  1 tbsp seafood seasoning or Old Bay seasoning
  1 tsp Worcestershire sauce
  1 tbsp light mayonnaise
  1/2 tsp baking powder
  2 lb fresh crabmeat

Combine egg, breadcrumbs, seafood seasoning, Worcestershire sauce, mayonnaise and baking powder in a large bowl. Stir in crabmeat. Mix well. Shape mixture into 8 one-half inch thick patties. Broil for 10 minutes without turning.

Eat two crab cakes for a single serving (refrigerate or freeze the rest for later consumption) and serve with 1 cup of any of the following steamed vegetables: asparagus, broccoli, eggplant, green beans, kale, snow pea pods, or spinach.

1800 CALORIES

Week 3 * Day 4

BREAKFAST: One cup of cereal (see cereal choices) and one cup soy milk or low-fat or skim milk, and one of the following: banana; apple; pear; 2 cups of strawberries (no sugar added); 1.5 cups of blueberries (no sugar added); 2 cups of raspberries (no sugar added); or low-calorie yogurt (100 calories).

MID-MORNING SNACK: Snacks may consist of two of the following choices: banana; apple; pear; 2 cups strawberries (no sugar added); 1.5 cups blueberries (no sugar added); 2 cups raspberries (no sugar added); low-calorie yogurt (100 calories); 1 oz of soy nuts (100 calories total, varies based on brand and preparation); 1 oz soy chips (I recommend Revival brand soy chips. Three to four times a week, if desired, you may substitute any 200-calorie food you desire, for example two part-skim mozzarella cheese sticks or 2 oz of chocolate (200 calories).

LUNCH: Shrimp and Avocado Sandwich Wrap
   8" whole-wheat tortilla wrap
   6 oz shrimp, fresh or frozen
   1/2 cup avocado, mashed

MID-AFTERNOON SNACK: Same as mid-morning snack.

DINNER: Gingered Beef and Broccoli, with rice.

Family size (serves 4)
   2 cups broccoli (keep stems 1/4 inch)
   1 cup cut snow peas
   1 red pepper, cut in half-inch pieces
   1/2 cup shitake mushrooms
   1 1/2 lb lean beef, cut for stir-fry
   3 tbsp water
   1 1/2 tbsp cornstarch
   2 tbsp olive oil
   1 tbsp fresh ginger, minced
   3/4 cup low-sodium soy sauce

Single serving
   1/4 of the above recipe (save the rest in refrigerator).

Add to a bowl the water, cornstarch, and soy sauce. Microwave broccoli, covered, on high power for 3 minutes. Heat nonstick skillet on high. When hot, pour 1 tsp olive oil into pan. Add ginger and beef and stir-fry until beef browns. Add sauce and toss to coat. Remove beef from pan. Add remaining oil. Add broccoli to pan along with peppers, mushrooms and snow peas. Stir-fry for 2 minutes. Return beef with sauce to pan, toss to evenly distribute.

Serve with 4 oz (half of a cup) of brown rice.

1800 CALORIES

Week 3 * Day 5

BREAKFAST: One cup of cereal (see cereal choices) and one cup soy milk or low-fat or skim milk, and one of the following: banana; apple; pear; 2 cups of strawberries (no sugar added); 1.5 cups of blueberries (no sugar added); 2 cups of raspberries (no sugar added); or low-calorie yogurt (100 calories).

MID-MORNING SNACK: Snacks may consist of two of the following choices: banana; apple; pear; 2 cups strawberries (no sugar added); 1.5 cups blueberries (no sugar added); 2 cups raspberries (no sugar added); low-calorie yogurt (100 calories); 1 oz of soy nuts (100 calories total, varies based on brand and preparation); 1 oz soy chips (I recommend Revival brand soy chips. Three to four times a week, if desired, you may substitute any 200-calorie food you desire, for example two part-skim mozzarella cheese sticks or 2 oz of chocolate (200 calories).

LUNCH: BBQ Pork Wrap
   8" whole-wheat tortilla wrap
   1 tsp onion powder
   2 tsp BBQ sauce
   2 tomato slices
   4 lettuce leaves
   6 oz pork loin

MID-AFTERNOON SNACK: Same as mid-morning snack.

DINNER: Lemon Baked Chicken, with rice and vegetable.

Family size (serves 4)	Single serving
Olive oil cooking spray	Olive oil cooking spray
2 tbsp fresh lemon juice	2 tsp fresh lemon juice
2 tbsp canola oil	2 tsp canola oil
1 clove of garlic, crushed	1/4 clove garlic, crushed
1/2 tsp fresh ground pepper	fresh ground pepper to taste
2 1/2 lbs boneless, sk inless chicken breasts	10 oz boneless, skinless chicken breast

Preheat oven to 350 degrees. Lightly spray a baking pan or a shallow casserole dish with cooking spray. In a small bowl, combine lemon juice, oil, garlic and pepper. Set aside. Rinse chicken and pat dry. Arrange chicken in prepared pan or dish. Pour lemon mixture over chicken pieces. Cover and bake for 40 minutes, or until tender, basting occasionally. Uncover and bake 10 minutes longer to allow chicken to brown.

Serve with 6 oz (3/4 cup) of cooked brown or wild rice and 1 cup of any of the following steamed vegetables asparagus, broccoli, eggplant, green beans, kale, snow pea pods, or spinach.

1800 CALORIES

Week 3 * Day 6

BREAKFAST: One cup of cereal (see cereal choices) and one cup soy milk or low-fat or skim milk, and one of the following: banana; apple; pear; 2 cups of strawberries (no sugar added); 1.5 cups of blueberries (no sugar added); 2 cups of raspberries (no sugar added); or low-calorie yogurt (100 calories).

MID-MORNING SNACK: Snacks may consist of two of the following choices: banana; apple; pear; 2 cups strawberries (no sugar added); 1.5 cups blueberries (no sugar added); 2 cups raspberries (no sugar added); low-calorie yogurt (100 calories); 1 oz of soy nuts (100 calories total, varies based on brand and preparation); 1 oz soy chips (I recommend Revival brand soy chips. Three to four times a week, if desired, you may substitute any 200-calorie food you desire, for example two part-skim mozzarella cheese sticks or 2 oz of chocolate (200 calories).

LUNCH: Island Wrap
   8" whole-wheat tortilla wrap
   2 lettuce leaves
   6 oz ham
   3 slices tomato
   1 tsp bacon bits
   1 oz mozzarella cheese
   1 oz pineapple
   2 tsp fat-free ranch dressing

MID-AFTERNOON SNACK: Same as mid-morning snack.

DINNER: Spinach Stuffed Sirloin

Family size (serves 4)	Single serving
2 1/2 lb lean sirloin steak, 1" to 1 1/2" thick	10 oz lean sirloin steak, 1" to 1 1/2" thick
1- 10 oz pkg frozen spinach, thawed and drained	4 oz pkg frozen spinach, thawed and drained
2 cloves garlic, crushed	1/2 clove garlic, crushed
cooking oil spray	cooking oil spray
1/4 lb mushrooms, finely chopped	2 oz mushrooms, finely chopped
1/2 cup diced red bell pepper (optional)	2 oz diced red bell pepper (optional)
1 tbsp olive oil	1 tsp olive oil
1/4 cup grated Parmesan cheese	1 oz grated Parmesan cheese

Preheat broiler. Meanwhile, heat oil in small sauté pan until hot but not smoking. Cook garlic, mushroom, and red bell pepper until softened. Add spinach and heat through. Stir in grated Parmesan thoroughly and remove from heat. With a sharp knife, cut pocket in sirloin steak nearly to the edges. Stuff with warm spinach mixture and place on rack in shallow pan. For medium rare, broil for 5 minutes on first side and 3 minutes, approximately, after turning steak over. For other doneness, adjust broiling time accordingly.

Serve with 6 oz (3/4 cup) of cooked brown or wild rice and 1 cup of any of the following steamed vegetables asparagus, broccoli, eggplant, green beans, kale, snow pea pods, or spinach.

1800 CALORIES

Week 3 * Day 7

BREAKFAST: One cup of cereal (see cereal choices) and one cup soy milk or low-fat or skim milk, and one of the following: banana; apple; pear; 2 cups of strawberries (no sugar added); 1.5 cups of blueberries (no sugar added); 2 cups of raspberries (no sugar added); or low-calorie yogurt (100 calories).

MID-MORNING SNACK: Snacks may consist of two of the following choices: banana; apple; pear; 2 cups strawberries (no sugar added); 1.5 cups blueberries (no sugar added); 2 cups raspberries (no sugar added); low-calorie yogurt (100 calories); 1 oz of soy nuts (100 calories total, varies based on brand and preparation); 1 oz soy chips (I recommend Revival brand soy chips. Three to four times a week, if desired, you may substitute any 200-calorie food you desire, for example two part-skim mozzarella cheese sticks or 2 oz of chocolate (200 calories).

LUNCH: BBQ Pork Burrito

8" whole-wheat tortilla wrap	1 oz low-fat mozzarella cheese
3 lettuce leaves	3 oz black beans
4 oz chicken	1 tsp barbeque sauce
3 tomato slices	1 tsp sour cream
1 oz corn	

MID-AFTERNOON SNACK: Same as mid-morning snack.

DINNER: Chicken Manicotti, with rice and vegetable.

Family size (serves 4)	Single serving
3/4 tsp oregano	1/4 tsp oregano
1/2 tsp marjoram	1 pinch marjoram
3/4 tsp sweet basil	1/4 tsp sweet basil
1/4 tsp fresh ground pepper	1 pinch fresh ground pepper
1- 6 oz can no-salt-added tomato paste	2 oz can no-salt-added tomato past
1 cup water	2 oz water
1 clove garlic, minced	1/4 clove garlic, minced
4 boneless, skinless chicken breasts, (about 2 1/2 lb), fat removed	1 boneless, skinless chicken breast, (10 oz), fat removed
4 oz low-fat cottage cheese, drained	1 oz low-fat cottage cheese, drained
2 oz grated part-skim mozzarella cheese	1 oz grated part-skim mozzarella

Preheat oven 350 degrees. In a small bowl, combine first four spices. Mix well. Set aside. In a small saucepan, blend tomato paste, water, and garlic. Add 3/4 of the seasoning mixture to the pan. Bring to a boil. Reduce heat and simmer 10 minutes, stirring occasionally. Meanwhile, rinse chicken and pat dry. Place breast fillets in a plastic bag and pound to 1/4" thickness. Set aside in a small bowl, combine remaining spice mixture with cottage cheese. Spoon mixtures onto centers of chicken breasts, leaving a 1/2 inch edge all around. From narrow end, roll each breast, leaving a 1/2 inch edge all around. Spoon half of the tomato mixture into the bottom of a 10 x 6 inch baking dish. Arrange chicken roll on top, seam side down. Spoon remaining tomato mixture over the chicken rolls. Top with mozzarella cheese and bake about 45 minutes, or until golden brown.

Serve with 6 oz (3/4cup) of cooked brown or wild rice and 1 cup of any of the following steamed vegetables: asparagus, broccoli, eggplant, green beans, kale, snow pea pods, or spinach.

Part Four:
Supplemental Meals

This section provides simple-to-prepare meals for those of you who don't enjoy cooking or who just don't have much time to do it. These are delicious examples of popular meals that stay within the nutritional parameters of the North Star Diet with regard to calories, fiber, etc. but are quicker to prepare and serve. These meals include omelet rollups and a new Quaker Oatmeal product, both good alternatives for breakfast; simple salad and sandwich ideas for lunch; and for dinner there are mix-and-match options for grilled dinners and satisfying salads. In addition there are some pasta and pizza ideas for lunch or dinner.

Breakfast Alternative Meals
> 1200, 1400, and 1600 Calorie Diets
>
> 1800 Calorie Diet

Lunch Alternative Meals
> 1200 and 1400 Calorie Diets
>
> 1600 and 1800 Calorie Diets

Dinner Alternative Meals
> 1200 and 1400 Calorie Diets
>
> 1600 Calorie Diet
>
> 1800 Calorie Diet

Pasta/Pizza Alternative Meals
> 1200, 1400, and 1600 Calorie Diets
>
> 1800 Calorie Diet

Breakfast Alternatives For
1200, 1400 and 1600 Calorie Diets

I strongly recommend the daily consumption of a high-fiber cereal, with at least 8 grams of fiber per serving, because multiple studies have revealed weight-loss and weight-maintenance goals can be more easily reached when these cereals are used. Nevertheless, the omelet rollup and Quaker Weight Control Oatmeal are also excellent alternatives.

Breakfast Alternative # 1: Omelet Rollup

8" whole-wheat wrap/tortilla (should contain a minimum of 10 g fiber).
2 eggs or egg substitute equivalent, scrambled in a pan with olive oil spray
1/2 oz shredded, low-fat Monterey jack or other low-fat cheese
vegetables as desired: mushrooms, onions, green peppers, tomatoes, etc.

Combine eggs, cheese, and vegetables in the wrap/tortilla.

Breakfast Alternative # 2: Quaker Weight Control Oatmeal

1 serving Quaker Weight Control Oatmeal (banana bread or cinnamon)
1/2 cup non-fat milk or soy milk
1 medium-sized apple, sliced, or a medium-sized banana, sliced

Prepare oatmeal and add milk and fruit. Serve.

Breakfast Alternatives For
1800 Calorie Diet

I strongly recommend the daily consumption of a high-fiber cereal, with at least 8 grams of fiber per serving, because multiple studies have revealed that weight-loss and weight-maintenance goals can be more easily reached when these cereals are used. Nevertheless, the omelet rollup and Quaker Weight Control Oatmeal are also excellent alternatives.

Breakfast Alternative # 1: Omelet Rollup

8" whole-wheat wrap/tortilla (should contain a minimum of 10 g fiber).
2 eggs or egg substitute equivalent, scrambled in pan with olive oil spray
1/2 oz shredded, low-fat Monterey jack or other low-fat cheese
vegetables as desired: mushrooms, onions, green peppers, tomatoes, etc.

Combine eggs, cheese, and vegetables in the wrap/tortilla.

Serve with one of the following: banana; apple; pear; 2 cups strawberries (no sugar added); 1.5 cups blueberries (no sugar added); 2 cups raspberries (no sugar added); or low-calorie yogurt (100 calories).

Breakfast Alternative # 2: Quaker Weight Control Oatmeal

1 serving Quaker Weight Control Oatmeal (banana bread or cinnamon)
1/2 cup of non-fat milk or soy milk
1 medium-sized apple, sliced, or a medium-sized banana, sliced

Prepare oatmeal and add milk and fruit.

Serve with one of the following: banana; apple; pear; 2 cups strawberries (no sugar added); 1.5 cups blueberries (no sugar added); 2 cups raspberries (no sugar added); or low-calorie yogurt (100 calories).

Lunch Alternatives For 1200 and 1400 Calorie Diets

Lunch Alternative # 1: Sandwich

I strongly recommend the use of whole-wheat wraps/tortillas as they allow you to maximize the fiber content of a meal while mini mizing the caloric content. Nevertheless, if you do not enjoy wraps/ tortillas you may substitute whole-wheat bread, making any of the wrap recipes into a sandwich. I strongly recommend the use of Natural Ovens bread. Each slice contains 60 calories and 4 grams of fiber. The bread tastes best when toasted. Other breads may be substituted but they should contain a minimum of 4 grams of fiber in each slice and no more than 70 calories per slice.

Lunch Alternative # 2: Single Serving Salad

375 Calorie Salad
  3 cups spinach
  1 cup mixed greens or lettuce

  Meat/Fish/Tofu (choose one)
4 oz turkey (roasted or grilled)	4 oz tuna (grilled)
4 oz chicken (grilled or baked, skinless)	4 oz shrimp (grilled)
4 oz ham (lean, center-cut)	4 oz scallops (grilled)
4 oz pork (center-cut pork chops)	4 oz lobster (grilled)
4 oz lean beef (sirloin tip or round)	4 oz white fish (baked or grilled)
4 oz tofu	

  1 oz shredded cheese (your choice) or 1/2 oz nuts (pine, almonds, peanuts, cashews) or crumbled bacon

  Liberal amounts of any combination of: tomatoes, green peppers, mushrooms, onions, sprouts, asparagus, broccoli, green beans, carrots, kale, and/or snow pea pods

  Dressing (choose one)
    2 tbsp Zero dressing, low-calorie
    2 tbsp flavored vinegar
    2 tbsp ranch, fat-free
    2 tbsp Italian, fat-free
    2 tbsp vinaigrette, low-calorie

Combine ingredients, toss and serve.

Lunch Alternatives For 1600 and 1800 Calorie Diets

Lunch alternative # 1: Sandwich

I strongly recommend the use of whole-wheat wraps/tortillas as they allow you to maximize the fiber content of a meal while minimizing the caloric content. Nevertheless, if you do not enjoy wraps/ tortillas you may substitute whole-wheat bread, making any of the wrap recipes into a sandwich. I strongly recommend the use of Natural Ovens bread. Each slice contains 60 calories and 4 grams of fiber. The bread tastes best when toasted. Other breads may be substituted but they should contain a minimum of 4 grams of fiber in each slice and no more than 70 calories per slice.

Lunch Alternative # 2: Single Serving Salad

475 Calorie Salad
  3 cups spinach
  1 cup mixed greens or lettuce

  Meat/Fish/Tofu (choose one):
      6 oz turkey (roasted or grilled)   6 oz tuna (grilled)
      6 oz chicken (grilled or baked, skinless) 6 oz shrimp (grilled)
      6 oz ham (lean, center-cut)   6 oz scallops (grilled)
      6 oz pork (center-cut pork chops)   6 oz lobster (grilled)
      6 oz lean beef (sirloin tip or round)   6 oz white fish (baked or grilled)
      6 oz tofu

  1 oz shredded cheese (your choice) or 1/2 oz nuts (pine, almonds, peanuts, cashews) or crumbled bacon

  Liberal amounts of any combination of: tomatoes, green peppers, mushrooms, onions, sprouts, asparagus, broccoli, green beans, carrots, kale, and/or snow pea pods

  Dressings (choose one)
      2 tbsp Zero dressing, low-calorie
      2 tbsp flavored vinegar
      2 tbsp ranch, fat-free
      2 tbsp Italian, fat-free
      2 tbsp vinaigrette, low-calorie

Combine ingredients, toss and serve.

Dinner Alternatives for 1200 and 1400 Calorie Diets

Dinner Alternative #1: Simplified Grilled Dinner

Meat/Fish/Tofu (choose one):

5 oz turkey (roasted or grilled)

5 oz chicken (grilled or baked, skinless)

5 oz ham (lean, center-cut)

5 oz pork (center-cut pork chops)

5 oz lean beef (sirloin tip or round)

5 oz tofu

5 oz tuna (grilled)

5 oz shrimp (grilled)

5 oz scallops (grilled)

5 oz lobster (grilled)

5 oz white fish (baked or grilled)

Seasonings (choose from list on next page)

Grill or broil protein portions with seasonings.

Serve with 3/4 cup of cooked brown rice or a 6 oz baked potato with skin, with butter buds or 2 sprays of butter-flavored spray and with 1 cup of any of the following steamed vegetables asparagus, broccoli, eggplant, green beans, kale, snow pea pods, or spinach.

Dinner Alternative # 2: Single Serving Salad

375 Calorie Salad

3 cups Spinach

1 cup mixed greens or lettuce

Meat/Fish/Tofu (choose one):

4 oz turkey (roasted or grilled)

4 oz chicken (grilled or baked, skinless)

4 oz ham (lean, center-cut)

4 oz pork (center-cut pork chops)

4 oz lean beef (sirloin tip or round)

4 oz tofu

4 oz tuna (grilled)

4 oz shrimp (grilled)

4 oz scallops (grilled)

4 oz lobster (grilled)

4 oz white fish (baked or grilled)

1 oz shredded cheese (your choice) or 1/2 oz nuts (pine, almonds, peanuts, cashews) or bacon, crumbled

Liberal amounts of: tomatoes, green peppers, mush rooms, onions, sprouts, asparagus, broccoli, green beans, carrots, kale, and/or snow pea pods

Dressings (choose one)

2 tbsp Zero dressing, low-calorie

2 tbsp ranch, fat-free

2 tbsp flavored vinegar

2 tbsp vinaigrette, low-calorie

2 tbsp Italian, fat-free

Combine ingredients, toss and serve.

Spices and Seasonings

The following spices may be utilized in any of the wraps or meals. Spices from most manufacturers contain no calories and may be applied as desired. Individuals with salt-restrictive diets or hypertension should utilize salt-free seasonings.

Garlic and Onion

California Style Crushed Garlic
California Style Garlic Salt
California Style Minced Garlic
California Style Onion Plus
California Style Onion
Garlic & Herb Spread
Garlic Bread Sprinkle
Garlic Powder
Garlic Spread
Minced Onions
Onion Powder

Wet California Style Garlic Powder
California Style Lemon & Pepper
Wet California Style Minced Onion
California Style Onion Powder
Salt Chopped Onions
Garlic & Parsley Salt
Garlic Juice
Garlic Salt
Minced Garlic
Onion Juice
Onion Salt

Seasoning Blends

Barbecue Seasoning
Cajun Seasoning
Caribbean Jerk Seasoning
Chicken Seasoning
Creole Seasoning
Garlic Pepper Blend
Herb Chicken Seasoning
Hot Shot!® Black & Red Pepper Blend
Lemon & Pepper Seasoning Salt
Mexican Seasoning
Rotisserie Chicken Seasoning
Salt'n Spice
Season-All® Seasoned Salt
Szechuan Style Pepper Blend

Broiled Steak Seasoning
California Style Garlic Pepper
Celery Salt
Classic Pizza Seasoning
Fajita Seasoning
Garlic Season-All® Seasoned Salt
Hickory Smoked Salt
Imitation Butter Flavor Salt
Mesquite Chicken Seasoning
Peppered Season-All Seasoned Salt
Salad Supreme Seasoning
Seafood Seasoning
Spicy Season-All® Seasoned Salt
Vegetable Supreme Seasoning

Herbs

Basil Leaves
Chives
Dill Weed
Ground Oregano
Ground Thyme
Marjoram Leaves
Parsley Flakes
Rubbed Sage
Tarragon Leaves

Bay Leaves
Cilantro Leaves
Ground Marjoram
Ground Sage
Italian Seasoning
Oregano Leaves
Rosemary Leaves
Sage Leaves
Thyme Leaves

Salt Free

Salt-Free All Purpose
Salt-Free It's a Dilly®
Salt-Free Spicy Seasoning

Salt-Free Garlic & Herb Seasoning
Salt-Free Lemon & Pepper Seasoning
Saltless Salt Substitute

Dinner Alternatives for 1600 Calorie Diet

Dinner Alternative # 1: Simplified Grilled Dinner

Meat/Fish/Tofu (choose one)
7 oz turkey (roasted or grilled)
7 oz chicken (grilled or baked, skinless)
7 oz ham (lean, center-cut)
7 oz pork (center-cut pork chops)
7 oz lean beef (sirloin tip or round)
7 oz tofu

7 oz tuna (grilled)
7 oz shrimp (grilled)
7 oz scallops (grilled)
7 oz lobster (grilled)
7 oz white fish (baked or grilled)

Seasonings (choose from list on next page)

Grill or broil protein portions with seasonings.

Serve with 3/4 cup of cooked brown rice or a 6 oz baked potato with skin, with butter buds or sprays of butter flavored spray, and with 1 cup of any of the following steamed vegetables asparagus, broccoli, eggplant, green beans, kale, snow pea pods, or spinach.

Dinner Alternative # 2: Single Serving Salad

475 Calorie Salad
3 cups spinach
1 cup mixed greens or lettuce

Meat/Fish/Tofu (choose one)
7 oz turkey (roasted or grilled)
7 oz chicken (grilled or baked, skinless)
7 oz ham (lean, center-cut)
7 oz pork (center-cut pork chops)
7 oz lean beef (sirloin tip or round)
7 oz tofu

7 oz tuna (grilled)
7 oz shrimp (grilled)
7 oz scallops (grilled)
7 oz lobster (grilled)
7 oz white fish (baked or grilled)

1 oz shredded cheese (your choice) or 1/2 oz nuts (pine, almonds, peanuts, cashews,) bacon crumbled

Liberal amounts of: tomatoes, green peppers, mushrooms, onions, sprouts, asparagus, broccoli, green beans, carrots, kale, and/or snow pea pods

Dressings (choose one)
2 tbsp Zero dressing, low-calorie
2 tbsp favored vinegar
2 tbsp vinaigrette, low-calorie

2 tbsp ranch, fat-free
2 tbsp Italian, fat-free

Combine ingredients, toss and serve.

Spices and Seasonings

The following spices may be utilized in any of the wraps or meals. Spices from most manufacturers contain no calories and may be applied as desired. Individuals with salt-restrictive diets or hypertension should utilize salt-free seasonings.

Garlic and Onion

California Style Crushed Garlic
California Style Garlic Salt
California Style Minced Garlic
California Style Onion Plus
California Style Onion
Garlic & Herb Spread
Garlic Bread Sprinkle
Garlic Powder
Garlic Spread
Minced Onions
Onion Powder

Wet California Style Garlic Powder
California Style Lemon & Pepper
Wet California Style Minced Onion
California Style Onion Powder
Salt Chopped Onions
Garlic & Parsley Salt
Garlic Juice
Garlic Salt
Minced Garlic
Onion Juice
Onion Salt

Seasoning Blends

Barbecue Seasoning
Cajun Seasoning
Caribbean Jerk Seasoning
Chicken Seasoning
Creole Seasoning
Garlic Pepper Blend
Herb Chicken Seasoning
Hot Shot!® Black & Red Pepper Blend
Lemon & Pepper Seasoning Salt
Mexican Seasoning
Rotisserie Chicken Seasoning
Salt'n Spice
Season-All® Seasoned Salt
Szechuan Style Pepper Blend

Broiled Steak Seasoning
California Style Garlic Pepper
Celery Salt
Classic Pizza Seasoning
Fajita Seasoning
Garlic Season-All® Seasoned Salt
Hickory Smoked Salt
Imitation Butter Flavor Salt
Mesquite Chicken Seasoning
Peppered Season-All Seasoned Salt
Salad Supreme Seasoning
Seafood Seasoning
Spicy Season-All® Seasoned Salt
Vegetable Supreme Seasoning

Herbs

Basil Leaves
Chives
Dill Weed
Ground Oregano
Ground Thyme
Marjoram Leaves
Parsley Flakes
Rubbed Sage
Tarragon Leaves

Bay Leaves
Cilantro Leaves
Ground Marjoram
Ground Sage
Italian Seasoning
Oregano Leaves
Rosemary Leaves
Sage Leaves
Thyme Leaves

Salt Free

Salt-Free All Purpose
Salt-Free It's a Dilly®
Salt-Free Spicy Seasoning

Salt-Free Garlic & Herb Seasoning
Salt-Free Lemon & Pepper Seasoning
Saltless Salt Substitute

Dinner Alternatives for 1800 Calorie Diet

Dinner Alternative # 1: Simplified Grilled Dinner

Meat/Fish/Tofu (choose one)
8 oz turkey (roasted or grilled)
8 oz chicken (grilled or baked, skinless)
8 oz ham (lean, center-cut)
8 oz pork (center-cut pork chops)
8 oz lean beef (sirloin tip or round)
8 oz tofu

8 oz tuna (grilled)
8 oz shrimp (grilled)
8 oz scallops (grilled)
8 oz lobster (grilled)
8 oz white fish (baked or grilled)

Seasonings (choose from list on next page)

Grill or broil portions with seasonings. Serve with 1 cup of cooked brown rice or a 7 oz baked potato with skin, with butter buds or 2 sprays of butter flavored spray, and with 1 cup of any of the following steamed vegetables: asparagus, broccoli, eggplant, green beans, kale, snow pea pods, or spinach.

Dinner Alternative # 2: Single Serving Salad

575 Calorie Salad
3 cups spinach
1 cup mixed greens or lettuce

Meat/Fish/Tofu (choose one):
8 oz turkey (roasted or grilled)
8 oz chicken (grilled or baked, skinless)
8 oz ham (lean, center-cut)
8 oz pork (center-cut pork chops)
8 oz lean beef (sirloin tip or round)
8 oz tofu

8 oz tuna (grilled)
8 oz shrimp (grilled)
8 oz scallops (grilled)
8 oz lobster (grilled)
8 oz white fish (baked or grilled)

2 oz shredded cheese (your choice) or 1 oz nuts (pine, almonds, peanuts, cashews) or bacon crumbled.

Liberal amounts of: tomatoes, green peppers, mushrooms, onions, sprouts, asparagus, broccoli, green beans, carrots, kale, and/or snow pea pods

Dressings (choose one):
2 tbsp Zero dressing, low-calorie
2 tbsp favored vinegar
2 tbsp vinaigrette, low-calorie

2 tbsp ranch, fat-free
2 tbsp Italian, fat-free

Combine ingredients, toss and serve.

Spices and Seasonings

The following spices may be utilized in any of the wraps or meals. Spices from most manufacturers contain no calories and may be applied as desired. Individuals with salt-restrictive diets or hypertension should utilize salt-free seasonings.

Garlic and Onion

California Style Crushed Garlic
California Style Garlic Salt
California Style Minced Garlic
California Style Onion Plus
California Style Onion
Garlic & Herb Spread
Garlic Bread Sprinkle
Garlic Powder
Garlic Spread
Minced Onions
Onion Powder

Wet California Style Garlic Powder
California Style Lemon & Pepper
Wet California Style Minced Onion
California Style Onion Powder
Salt Chopped Onions
Garlic & Parsley Salt
Garlic Juice
Garlic Salt
Minced Garlic
Onion Juice
Onion Salt

Seasoning Blends

Barbecue Seasoning
Cajun Seasoning
Caribbean Jerk Seasoning
Chicken Seasoning
Creole Seasoning
Garlic Pepper Blend
Herb Chicken Seasoning
Hot Shot!® Black & Red Pepper Blend
Lemon & Pepper Seasoning Salt
Mexican Seasoning
Rotisserie Chicken Seasoning
Salt'n Spice
Season-All® Seasoned Salt
Szechuan Style Pepper Blend

Broiled Steak Seasoning
California Style Garlic Pepper
Celery Salt
Classic Pizza Seasoning
Fajita Seasoning
Garlic Season-All® Seasoned Salt
Hickory Smoked Salt
Imitation Butter Flavor Salt
Mesquite Chicken Seasoning
Peppered Season-All Seasoned Salt
Salad Supreme Seasoning
Seafood Seasoning
Spicy Season-All® Seasoned Salt
Vegetable Supreme Seasoning

Herbs

Basil Leaves
Chives
Dill Weed
Ground Oregano
Ground Thyme
Marjoram Leaves
Parsley Flakes
Rubbed Sage
Tarragon Leaves

Bay Leaves
Cilantro Leaves
Ground Marjoram
Ground Sage
Italian Seasoning
Oregano Leaves
Rosemary Leaves
Sage Leaves
Thyme Leaves

Salt Free

Salt-Free All Purpose
Salt-Free It's a Dilly®
Salt-Free Spicy Seasoning

Salt-Free Garlic & Herb Seasoning
Salt-Free Lemon & Pepper Seasoning
Saltless Salt Substitute

Pasta Lunch or Dinner For 1200 or 1400 Calorie Diets

Pasta Lunch or Dinner

375 Calorie Pasta Meal

2 oz (3/4 cup) dry whole-wheat pasta (Favorite varieties: Ronzoni Healthy Harvest, Barilla Plus Pasta, and Revival Soy Pasta).

1/2 cup red sauce (Favorites: Classico Four Cheese, and Bertolli Tomato Basil. No white sauce substitutions).

Meat/Fish/Tofu (choose one):

2 oz turkey (roasted or grilled)	2 oz tuna (grilled)
2 oz chicken (grilled or baked, skinless)	2 oz shrimp (grilled)
2 oz ham (lean, center-cut)	2 oz scallops (grilled)
2 oz pork (center-cut pork chops)	2 oz lobster (grilled)
2 oz lean beef (sirloin tip or round)	2 oz white fish (baked or grilled)
2 oz tofu	

Cook pasta al dente. Add red sauce and protein choice. Top with a sprinkle of grated Parmesan cheese and serve.

Pasta Lunch or Dinner
for 1600 Calorie Diet

Pasta Lunch or Dinner

475 Calorie Pasta Meal

2 1/2 oz (1 cup) dry whole-wheat pasta (favorite varieties: Ronzoni Healthy Harvest, Barilla Plus Pasta, and Revival Soy Pasta).

1/2 cup red sauce (favorites: Classico Four Cheese and Bertolli Tomato Basil. No white sauce substitutions).

Meat/Fish/Tofu (choose one):
- 3 oz turkey (roasted or grilled)
- 3 oz chicken (grilled or baked, skinless)
- 3 oz ham (lean, center-cut)
- 3 oz pork (center-cut pork chops)
- 3 oz lean beef (sirloin tip or round)
- 3 oz tofu
- 3 oz tuna (grilled)
- 3 oz shrimp (grilled)
- 3 oz scallops (grilled)
- 3 oz lobster (grilled)
- 3 oz white fish (baked or grilled)

Cook pasta al dente. Add red sauce and protein choice. Top with a sprinkle of grated Parmesan cheese and serve.

Pasta Lunch or Dinner
for 1800 Calorie Diet

Pasta Lunch or Dinner

575 Calorie Pasta Meal

2 1/2 oz (1 cup) dry whole-wheat pasta (favorite varieties: Ronzoni Healthy Harvest, Barilla Plus Pasta, and Revival Soy Pasta).

1/2 cup red sauce (favorites: Classico Four Cheese and Bertolli Tomato Basil. No white sauce substitutions).

Meat/Fish/Tofu (choose one):
5 oz turkey (roasted or grilled)	5 oz tuna (grilled)
5 oz chicken (grilled or baked, skinless)	5 oz shrimp (grilled)
5 oz ham (lean, center-cut)	5 oz scallops (grilled)
5 oz pork (center-cut pork chops)	5 oz lobster (grilled)
5 oz lean beef (sirloin tip or round)	5 oz white fish (baked or grilled)
5 oz tofu	

Cook pasta al dente. Add red sauce and protein choice. Top with a sprinkle of grated Parmesan Cheese and serve.

Pizza Alternative for 1200, 1400 and 1600 Calorie Diets

Pizza Lunch or Dinner Alternative

2 Mission Brand, carb-balance, soft taco size tortillas
2 oz pizza sauce
3 oz low-fat, part-skim mozzarella cheese
thinly sliced vegetables, if desired

Bake tortillas at 375 degrees for approximately 3-5 minutes or until golden brown. Add pizza sauce and cheese. Divide toppings between tortillas. Cook for an additional 3-5 minutes until the cheese melts.

Pizza Alternative for 1800 Calorie Diet

Pizza Lunch or Dinner Alternative

3 Mission Brand, carb-balance, soft taco size tortillas
3 oz pizza sauce
4 1/2 oz low-fat, part-skim mozzarella cheese
thinly sliced vegetables, if desired

Bake tortillas at 375 degrees for approximately 3-5 minutes or until golden brown. Add pizza sauce and cheese. Divide toppings between tortillas. Cook for an additional 3-5 minutes until the cheese melts.

Part Five: North Star Diet, Progression Version

The progression version of the North Star Diet slowly implements dietary and lifestyle changes. It allows individuals to change their eating habits over a period of months. Each change is broken down into a series of small steps and is less overwhelming than a complete lifestyle overhaul all at once.

Step 1. Daily exercise.

A) Start by completing 10 minutes of moderate daily activity. Moderate activity is activity which can be completed while comfortably talking to another individual. Examples of potential activities: a brisk walk, riding a stationary bike or regular bike (weather permitting), a light run, swim or water aerobics.

B) Increase your daily activity level by 10 minutes each month for 6 months. At the end of 6 months you should be completing 60 minutes of moderate activity each day. Sixty minutes of moderate activity is also the equivalent of 10,000 steps a day. An easy way to determine if you're reaching this level is to use a pedometer. A pedometer is an inexpensive device which can be purchased at any sporting goods or department store and measures the number of steps, or up and down movements, in a given period.

C) Once you have reached the level of 60 minutes of daily activity you may choose to continue with 60 minutes of moderate activity or begin intensifying your efforts toward reaching the equivalent of 30 minutes of strenuous activity on a daily basis. This is a level of activity during which an individual could not comfortably carry on a conversation with another individual. An example of strenuous activity is a light jog. Moderate or strenuous activity can be completed in 10-minute blocks if desired. Your ultimate goal is to achieve either 60 minutes of moderate or 30 minutes of vigorous activity on a daily basis.

Step 2. Consume two liters of fluid a day, which is approximately 80 ounces. Eighty ounces of fluid is the equivalent of 8 ounces of water each hour for ten hours a day, or two 8-ounce glasses of water with each meal and snack. You may substitute diet soda pop or tea with meals if desired but no fruit juice or regular pop is allowed.

Step 3. One month after the initiation of daily exercise and two liters of daily fluid, start consuming a healthy breakfast. Breakfast options can be chosen from the calorie-specific meal plans and alternative meal plans found in Part Four and Part Five. Follow the calorie-specific guidelines for your current weight and gender. As you lose weight continue to select the appropriate breakfast level:

FEMALES

Weight in lbs	Caloric content of breakfast
≤250 lbs	250 calories based on a 1200 calorie diet
≥250 ≤300 lbs	250 calories based on a 1400 calorie diet
≥ 300 lbs	250 calories based on a 1600 calorie diet

MALES

Weight in lbs	Caloric content of breakfast
≤250 lbs	250 calories based on a 1400 calorie diet
≥250 ≤300 lbs	250 calories based on a 1600 calorie diet
≥ 300 lbs	350 calories based on a 1800 calorie diet

Step 4. One month following the initiation of an appropriate high-fiber breakfast, begin adding calorie-specific snacks, in the middle of the morning and in the middle of the afternoon. Follow the calorie-specific guidelines for your weight. As you lose weight continue to select the appropriate dietary plan. Both snacks may consist of one (1200-calorie plan) or two (1400, 1600, 1800 calorie plans) of the following choices: banana; apple; pear; 2 cups strawberries (no sugar added); 1.5 cups blueberries (no sugar added); 2 cups raspberries (no sugar added); low-calorie yogurt (100 calories); 1 oz of soy nuts (100 calories total, varies based on brand and preparation); 1 oz soy chips (I recommend Revival brand soy chips). Failure to eat timely mid-morning and mid-afternoon snacks will decrease your fat-burning capacity, or metabolism. Three to four times a week, if desired, you may substitute any food you desire (100 to 200 calories depending upon meal plan), for example a part-skim mozzarella cheese stick or 1 oz of chocolate (100 calories). Your snacks should be chosen from the following chart according to your current weight:

FEMALES

Weight in lbs	Caloric content of snacks, mid morning, mid afternoon
≤250 lbs	100 calorie snack based on a 1200 calorie diet
≥250 ≤300 lbs	200 calorie snack based on a 1400 calorie diet
≥ 300 lbs	200 calorie snack based on a 1600 calorie diet

MALES

Weight in lbs	Caloric content of snacks, mid morning, mid afternoon
≤250 lbs	200 calorie snack based on a 1400 calorie diet
≥250 ≤300 lbs	200 calorie snack based on a 1600 calorie diet
≥ 300 lbs	200 calorie snack based on a 1800 calorie diet

Step 5. One month following the initiation of calorie-specific healthy snacks twice a day, implement a calorie-specific healthy lunch. Lunch options can be chosen from the meal plans and alternate meal plans. Follow the caloric guidelines for your weight. As you lose weight continue to select the appropriate dietary lunch plan from the list below.

FEMALES

Weight in lbs	Caloric content of lunch
≤250 lbs	375 calories based on a 1200 calorie diet
≥250 ≤300 lbs	375 calories based on a 1400 calorie diet
≥ 300 lbs	475 calories based on a 1600 calorie diet

MALES

Weight in lbs	Caloric content of snacks, mid morning, mid afternoon
≤250 lbs	375 calories based on a 1400 calorie diet
≥250 ≤300 lbs	375 calories based on a 1600 calorie diet
≥ 300 lbs	475 calories based on a 1800 calorie diet

Step 6. One month following the initiation of a calorie-specific lunch, implement a calorie-specific healthy dinner. Dinner options can be chosen from the meal plans and alternate meal plans, Part Four and Part Five. Follow the caloric guidelines for your weight. As you lose weight continue to select the appropriate dinner plan for your current weight:

FEMALES

Weight in lbs	Caloric content of Dinner
≤250 lbs	375 calories based on a 1200 calorie diet
≥250 ≤300 lbs	375 calories based on a 1400 calorie diet
≥ 300 lbs	475 calories based on a 1600 calorie diet

MALES

Weight in lbs	Caloric content of Dinner
≤250 lbs	375 calories based on a 1400 calorie diet
≥250 ≤300 lbs	475 calories based on a 1600 calorie diet
≥ 300 lbs	575 calories based on a 1800 calorie diet

Step 7. Consume dinner 3-4 hours prior to bedtime. If you eat closer to bedtime there is an increased chance the food will be stored and converted into fat while you sleep. If you are still hungry after dinner, you may consume an apple, pear or banana or 1 oz of lean grilled protein: turkey, ham, beef, or fish.

Step 8. Consume a daily multi-vitamin, 1200 mg calcium carbonate, 1000 I.U. Vitamin D, and 1000-3000 mg fish oil.

Step 9. Consumption of two cups of green tea, one tea bag per cup, will promote 70 calories of weight loss on a daily basis. A personal favorite is Tazo Zen brand of green tea.

Step 10 . Once you have achieved your weight-loss goals, efforts should be directed at maintaining your desired weight. The North Star Diet and Weight Maintenance Program is greatly concerned with individuals achieving weight loss and maintaining their weight at a desired stable weight. The maintenance of a stable, non-fluctuating weight is dependent on two factors: 60-90 minutes of moderate daily exercise and accurate determination of the Resting Energy Expenditure (REE). Resting Energy Expenditure is the amount of daily energy, in calories, required to maintain an individual's weight. REE can be calculated by utilizing the Revised Harris-Benedict Equation, and multiplying the value by a coefficient which may be anywhere from 1.0 to 2.0.

Revised Harris-Benedict Equation

MALES
$66.5 + (6.25 \times lbs) + (12.7 \times inches) - (6.77 \times Age) = REE$

FEMALES
$665.1 + (4.34x\ lb) + (4.7 \times inches) - (4.676 \times Age) = REE$

> REE is expressed in calories per day.
> Height is expressed in inches.
> Weight is expressed in pounds.
> Age is expressed in years.

Once you have calculated your REE, I recommend that you start by multiplying the value by 1.2. Consume the calculated daily amount of calories for a week. If your weight decreases during that week you must adjust your intake upward. Multiply by 1.3 or 1.4, increasing your caloric consumption accordingly until your weight remains stable. The coefficient by which you multiply the REE will vary in each individual depending on the amount of exercise done on a daily basis, muscle mass, and fidgeting. Therefore, individuals who exercise more daily, have a greater muscle mass, or have a higher metabolism will have proportionally greater caloric requirements. Once, you have accurately determined your individual REE, attempt to consume the designated caloric level as this will help you maintain your desired weight.

Part Six:
North Star Weight Maintenance Guidelines

Adding exercise to your diet plan will aid you in maintaining the weight loss you have achieved through the use of the North Star Diet. The guidelines for the weight maintenance program are outlined below.

1) Daily exercise, consisting of both strength training and aerobic exercise.

2) Strength training will be completed for three consecutive days, followed by one day of rest. The three day strength training regimen will be completed twice in one week.

3) Aerobic exercise will be completed daily. Week #1 will consist of a minimum of 10 minutes of aerobic activity. The amount of aerobic activity should be increased by 10 minutes a week until 30 minutes is achieved. The aerobic activity may consist of a brisk walk, riding a stationary bike (or regular bike, weather permitting), a light run, swim or water aerobics.

4) Gradually increase strength training sessions with the ultimate goal of 6 days a week, with 30 minutes of aerobic activity daily, and on 1 day a week, 60 minutes of moderate activity (brisk walk) or 30 minutes of vigorous activity (light run or swim).

5) Many individuals may find the exercise goals listed above to be intimidating. If you want to begin an exercise program but at a slower pace, an alternate exercise regimen can be found at the end of this section.

Strength Training Rules

1) Strength training will be completed for 3 consecutive days followed by one day of rest. The strength training regimen will then be repeated. A total of six days of strength training will be completed on a weekly basis.

2) Start each strength training session with 15-20 modified jumping jacks (see Exercise Days 1-3, exercise #1).

3) Many of the strength exercises involve exercise bands for resistance. Resistance bands can be purchased in many sizes and resistances, at almost all sports stores and large department and discount merchants. Purchase resistance bands with the least amount of resistance. As you become stronger you should acquire resistance bands with increasing resistance. An excellent web site for exercise fitness bands is http://www.bodytrends.com/

4) Exercise equipment required to complete all exercises listed in Strength Training Days #1-3:

    a. Carpeted floor or exercise/yoga mat
    b. One fitness band
    c. Fitness figure-eight band
    d. Fitness band door attachment
    e. Aerobic step

5) Your goal is to complete 15-20 repetitions within each exercise. The last 4-5 repetitions within each exercise should produce a mild amount of resistance. If you are unable to complete the full 15-20 repetitions, attempt to complete 5 more repetitions beyond the point at which you begin to feel resistance.

6) Take a maximum of 2 minutes rest between each exercise. There are a total of eight strength training exercises to be completed each day. As your fitness level improves, decrease your rest time between each strength training exercise. We recommend that you decrease the time between each exercise by 15 seconds per week. The ultimate goal is to spend 1 minute or less between exercises. If you are able to limit your rest time to 30-60 seconds between exercises you will achieve maximal benefit. You will both build muscle, which will increase your metabolism, and elevate your heart rate to the same level achieved during a brisk walk.

7) To assist exercise compliance, you may utilize the exercise diary sheets found in the appendix. The first exercise sheet allows you to record the type of exercise and time spent. The second exercise sheet allows you to record the total steps completed in a given day with a pedometer. Goal of the step chart is to complete 10,000 steps a day.

Daily Exercise Chart

Week #1

Monday	Tuesday	Wednesday	Thursday	Friday	Saturday	Sunday
Day # 1 Strength Training	Day # 2 Strength Training	Day # 3 Strength Training		Day # 1 Strength Training	Day # 2 Strength Training	Day # 3 Strength Training
10 Minutes Aerobic Activity	10 Minutes Aerobic Activity	10 Minutes Aerobic Activity	20 Minutes Aerobic Activity	10 Minutes Aerobic Activity	10 Minutes Aerobic Activity	10 Minutes Aerobic Activity

Week #2

Monday	Tuesday	Wednesday	Thursday	Friday	Saturday	Sunday
Day # 1 Strength Training	Day # 2 Strength Training	Day # 3 Strength Training		Day # 1 Strength Training	Day # 2 Strength Training	Day # 3 Strength Training
20 Minutes Aerobic Activity	20 Minutes Aerobic Activity	20 Minutes Aerobic Activity	40 Minutes Aerobic Activity	20 Minutes Aerobic Activity	20 Minutes Aerobic Activity	20 Minutes Aerobic Activity

Week #3

Monday	Tuesday	Wednesday	Thursday	Friday	Saturday	Sunday
Day # 1 Strength Training	Day # 2 Strength Training	Day # 3 Strength Training		Day # 1 Strength Training	Day # 2 Strength Training	Day # 3 Strength Training
30 Minutes Aerobic Activity	30 Minutes Aerobic Activity	30 Minutes Aerobic Activity	60 Minutes Aerobic Activity	30 Minutes Aerobic Activity	30 Minutes Aerobic Activity	30 Minutes Aerobic Activity

Continue week #3 to achieve weight-maintenance goals.

DAY 1. Exercise #1: Jumping Jacks Warm-up

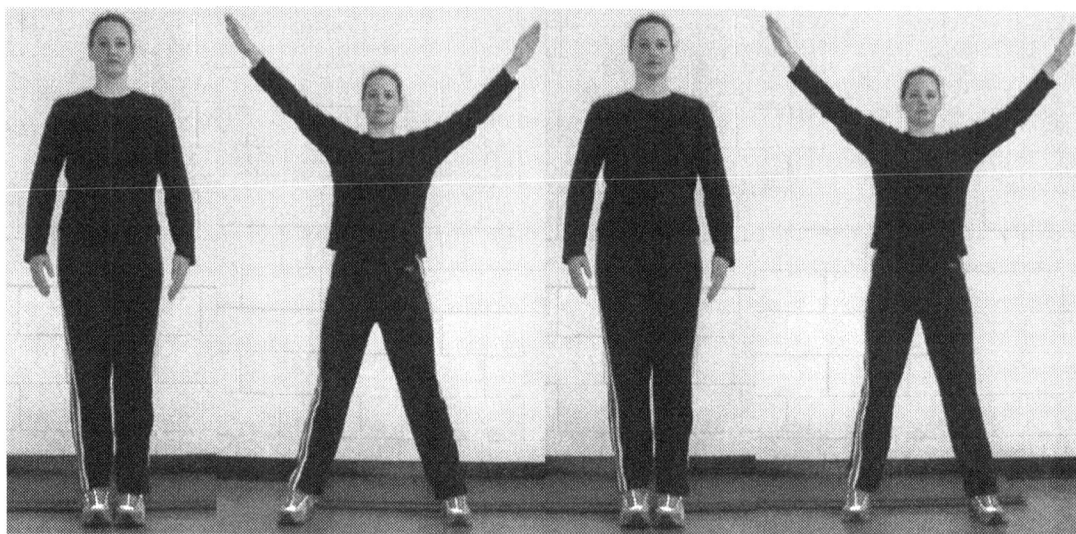

| Figure 1 | Figure 2 | Figure 3 | Figure 4 |

Muscles utilized: Shoulder, back, legs, butt.

Number of Repetitions: Goal of 15-20 repetitions, or if you are unable to complete the full 15-20 repetitions, attempt to complete 5 more repetitions beyond the point at which you begin to feel fatigue.

Modified Jumping Jacks:

Figure1. Start with legs together, standing comfortably.

Figure 2. Slide right leg outward to side while simultaneously raising both hands.

Figure 3. Return to a relaxed state.

Figure 4. Slide left leg while simultaneously raising both hands.

Rest for a maximum of 2 minutes before starting the next exercise. As your fitness level improves decrease your rest time between each strength training exercise. We recommend that you decrease the rest time between each exercise by 15 seconds a week. The goal is to have 1 minute or less between exercises.

DAY 1. Exercise #2: Squat

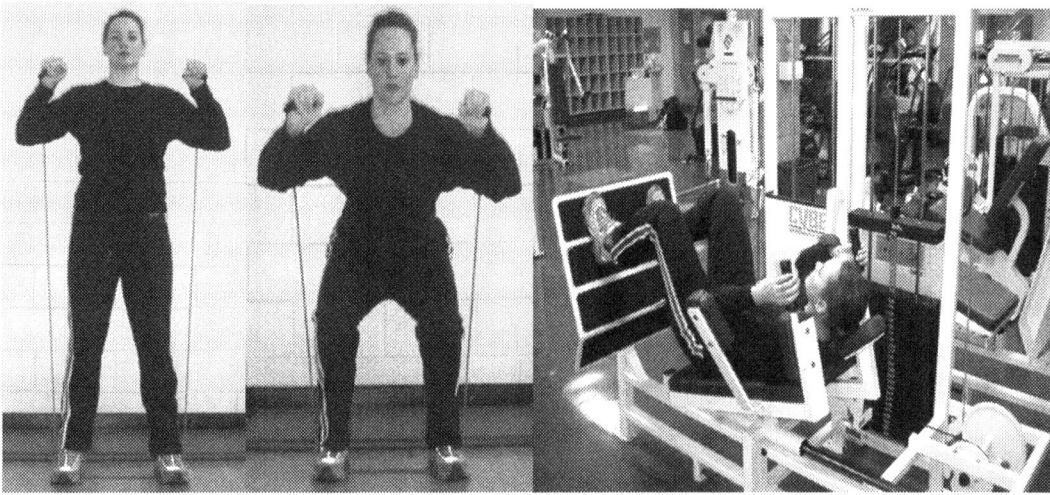

Figure 1   Figure 2   Figure 3

Muscles utilized: Legs, butt.

Number of Repetitions: Goal 15-20, or if you are unable to complete the full 15-20 repetitions, attempt to complete 5 more repetitions beyond the point at which you begin to feel resistance.

Figure 1. (Start) Place feet approximately shoulder-width apart in the center of the exercise band. Place the tube under the arch of each foot.

Figure 2. (Finish) Keep head up, back flat as you squat, bending the knees in a slow and controlled manner. Straighten knees to stand up.

Figure 3. Example of a squat utilizing a leg press in a gym.

Rest for a maximum of 2 minutes before starting the next exercise. As your fitness level improves decrease your rest time between each strength training exercise. We recommend that you decrease the rest time between each exercise by 15 seconds a week. The goal is to have 1 minute or less between exercises.

DAY 1. Exercise #3: Lateral Raise

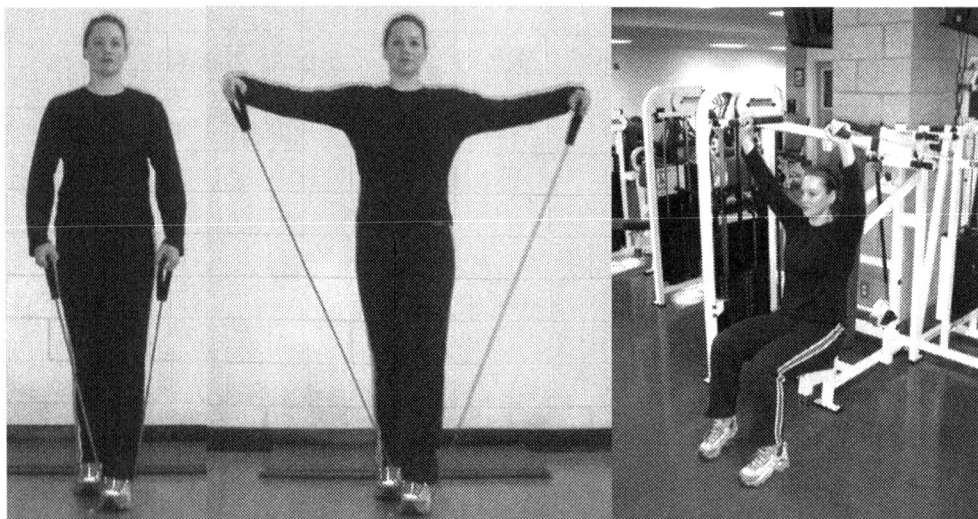

| Figure 1 | Figure 2 | Figure 3 |

Muscles utilized: Shoulder.

Number of Repetitions: Goal 15-20, or if you are unable to complete the full 15-20 repetitions, attempt to complete 5 more repetitions beyond the point at which you begin to feel resistance.

Figure 1. (Start) While standing, place the center of the exercise band under the arch of one foot. Grasp both handles and stand with arms down at your sides.

Figure 2. (Finish) Raise both arms laterally, out to your sides. Hold arms stationary when at shoulder height, palms should face the floor. Bring the arms back down to the start position in a slow, controlled manner.

Figure 3. Example of a deltoid press machine in a gym.

Rest for a maximum of 2 minutes before starting the next exercise. As your fitness level improves decrease your rest time between each strength training exercise. We recommend that you decrease the rest time between each exercise by 15 seconds a week. The goal is to have 1 minute or less between exercises.

DAY 1. Exercise # 4: Biceps Curl

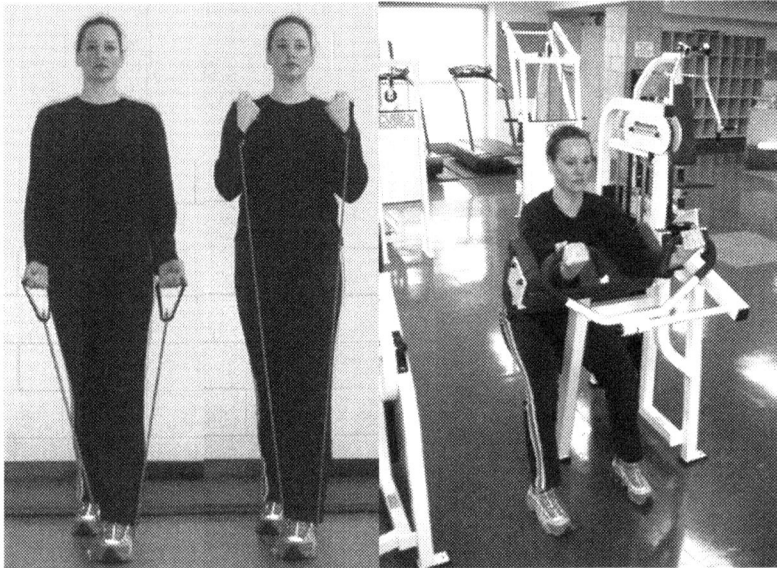

| Figure 1 | Figure 2 | Figure 3 |

Muscles utilized: Biceps, forearm.

Number of Repetitions: Goal 15-20, or if you are unable to complete the full 15-20 repetitions, attempt to complete 5 more repetitions beyond the point at which you begin to feel resistance.

Figure 1. (Start) Standing, place the center of the fitness tube securely under the arch of forward foot. Grasp one fitness tube handle in each hand and extend your arms at your side.

Figure 2. (Finish) Keeping your elbows at your sides, bend both elbows, taking care to bring your palms toward your body in the direction of your shoulders. Hold for a second. Extend your arms back down to the start position at your sides in a slow, controlled manner. Alternate feet and repeat.

Figure 3. Example of a bicep curl utilizing biceps machine.

Rest for a maximum of 2 minutes before starting the next exercise. As your fitness level improves decrease your rest time between each strength training exercise. We recommend that you decrease the rest time between each exercise by 15 seconds a week. The goal is to have 1 minute or less between exercises.

DAY 1. Exercise #5: Reverse Rows

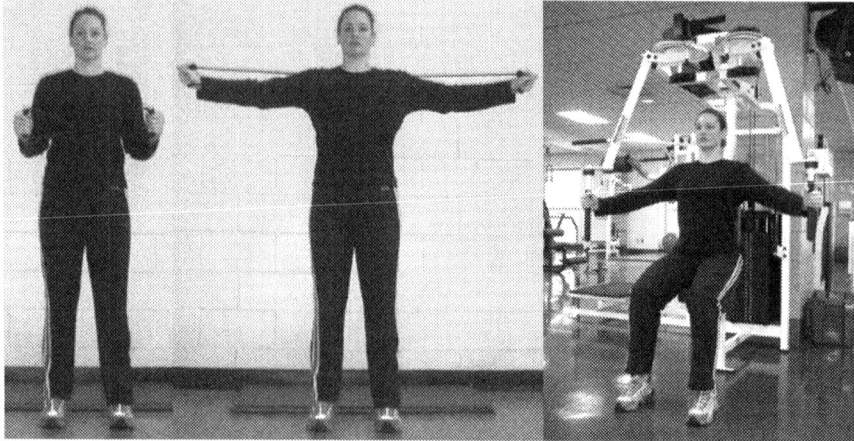

Figure 1   Figure 2   Figure 3

Muscles utilized: Upper and middle back and chest.

Number of Repetitions: Goal 15-20, or if you are unable to complete the full 15-20 repetitions, attempt to complete 5 more repeti tions beyond the point at which you begin to feel resistance.

Figure 1. (Start) Stand with erect posture, feet shoulder-width apart, and knees slightly bent. Grasp each handle of figure-8 band, and extend both arms out in front of the body at shoulder level.

Figure 2. (Finish) Pull your arms apart, laterally out to each side maintaining the arms up at shoulder height. Squeeze the shoulder blades together, pause briefly, and slowly bring both arms back to the start position, extended straight out in front of your body.

Figure 3. Example of incline press utilizing pectoral machine.

Rest for a maximum of 2 minutes before starting the next exercise. As your fitness level improves decrease your rest time between each strength training exercise. We recommend that you decrease the rest time between each exercise by 15 seconds a week. The goal is to have 1 minute or less between exercises.

DAY 1. Exercise # 6: Upper Back Extension

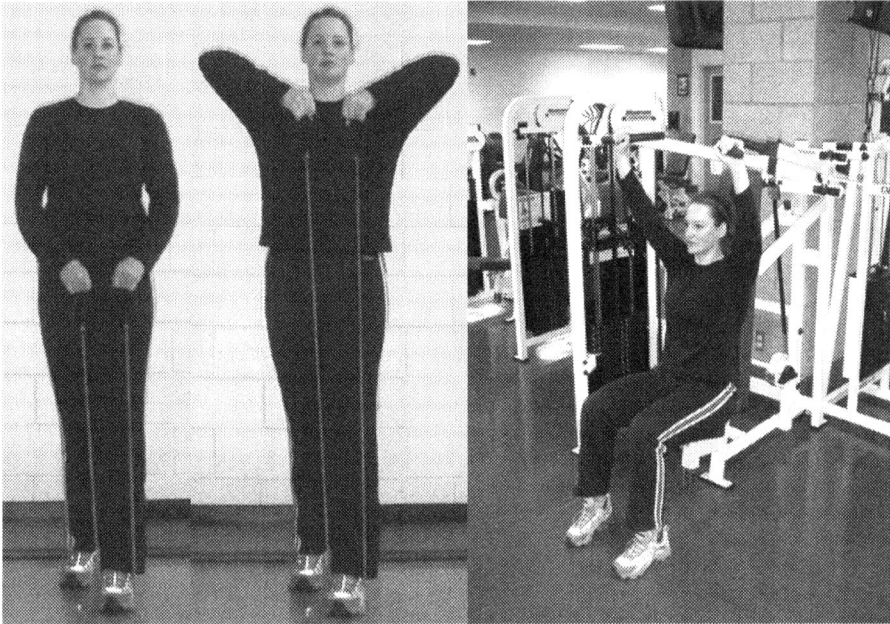

Figure 1   Figure 2   Figure 3

Muscles utilized: Upper and middle back and chest.

Number of Repetitions: Goal 15-20, or if you are unable to complete the full 15-20 repetitions, attempt to complete 5 more repetitions beyond the point at which you begin to feel resistance.

Figure 1. (Start) While standing, secure one of the exercise band handles under the arch of one foot and grab the opposite foam handle with both hands extended down in front of your body. Alternate feet and repeat.

Figure 2. (Finish) Leading with the elbows, raise both arms up and out to the sides, ending with both hands up under the chin as shown.

Figure 3. Example of a seated military press machine.

Rest for a maximum of 2 minutes before starting the next exercise. As your fitness level improves decrease your rest time between each strength training exercise. We recommend that you decrease the rest time between each exercise by 15 seconds a week. The goal is to have 1 minute or less between exercises.

DAY 1. Exercise #7: Standing Hip Abduction

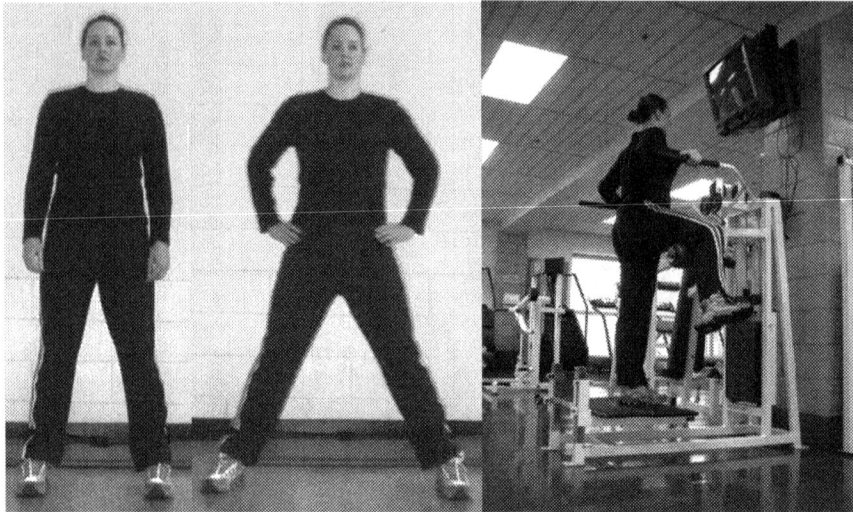

Figure 1   Figure 2   Figure 3

Muscles utilized: Outer thigh, inner thigh.

Number of Repetitions: Goal 15-20, or if you are unable to complete the full 15-20 repetitions, attempt to complete 5 more repetitions beyond the point at which you begin to feel resistance.

Figure 1. (Start) Place one foot into each of the loops formed by the figure-8 exercise band. Bring the figure-8 band up to position each foam handle just above each ankle. Stand with erect posture and feet about shoulder-width apart.

Figure 2. (Finish) Standing on one foot, step out laterally, with the opposite leg to the side of the body, stretching the figure 8 band far enough to form a wider than hip width stance. Bring the leg back to the start posi tion in a slow, controlled manner.

Figure 3. Example of adductor/abductor machine.

Rest for a maximum of 2 minutes before starting the next exercise. As your fitness level improves decrease your rest time between each strength training exercise. We recommend that you decrease the rest time between each exercise by 15 seconds a week. The goal is to have 1 minute or less between exercises.

DAY 1. Exercise # 8: Sit Ups

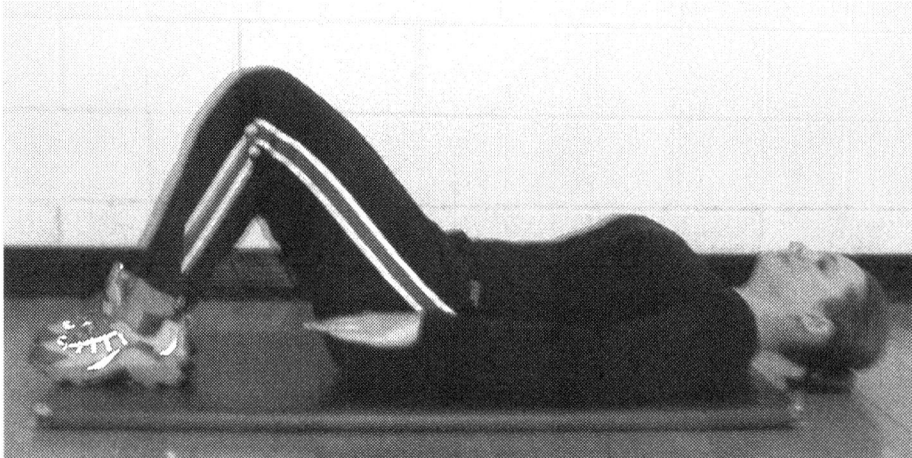

Figure 1

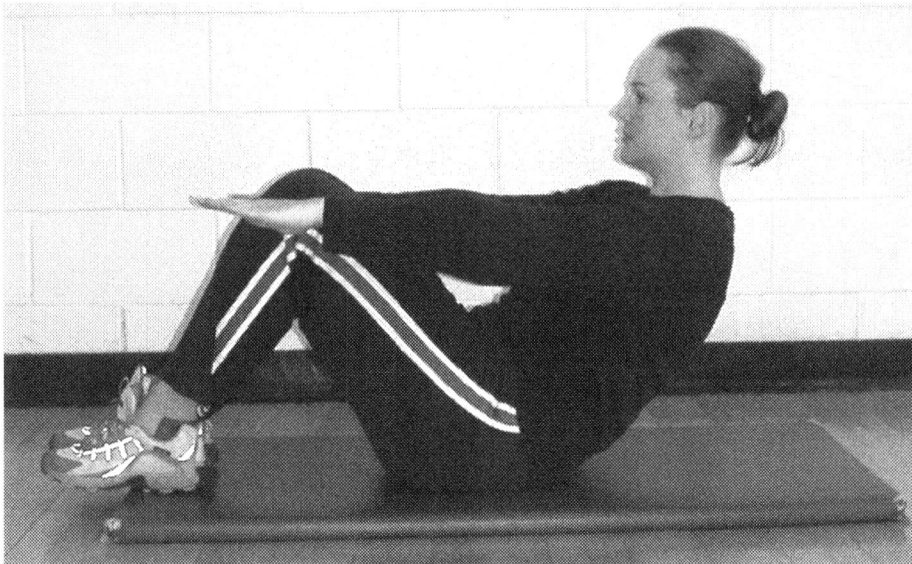

Figure 2

Muscles utilized: Abdominals.

Number of Repetitions: Goal 15-20, or if you are unable to complete the full 15-20 repetitions, attempt to complete 5 more repetitions beyond the point at which you begin to feel resistance.

Figure 1. (Start) Legs bent, lying on floor, arms to the side.

Figure 2. (Finish) Raise torso off the floor until hands extend to the knees, while keeping your feet firmly on the floor. Hold your position for one second, then slowly and gradually return your back to the floor.

Day 1 Exercise Review

Exercise # 1   Exercise # 2

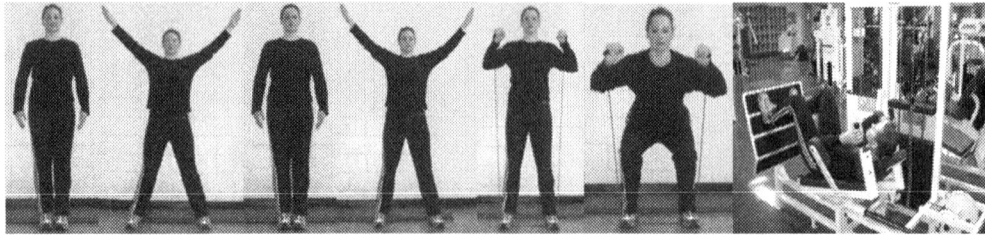

Fig 1   Fig 2   Fig 3   Fig 4   Fig 1   Fig 2   Fig 3

Exercise # 3   Exercise # 4

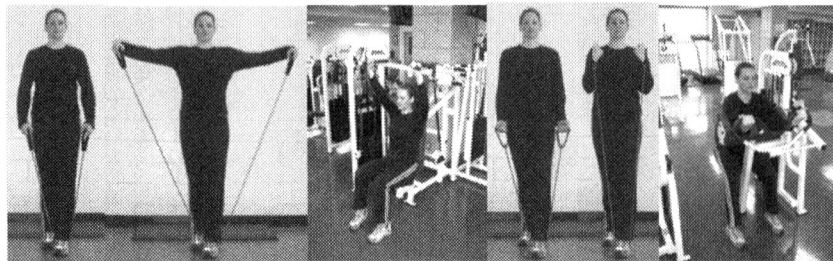

Fig 1   Fig 2   Fig 3   Fig 1   Fig 2   Fig 3

Exercise # 5   Exercise # 6

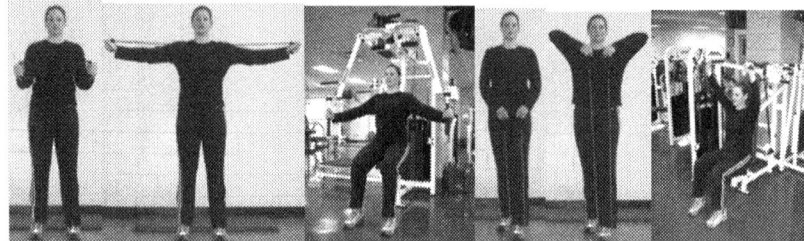

Fig 1   Fig 2   Fig 3   Fig 1   Fig 2   Fig 3

Exercise # 7   Exercise # 8

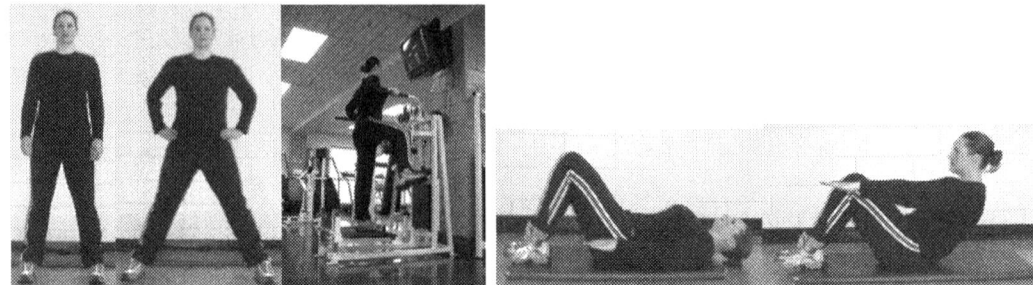

Fig 1   Fig 2   Fig 3   Fig 1   Fig 2

DAY 2. Exercise #1: Jumping Jacks Warm-Up

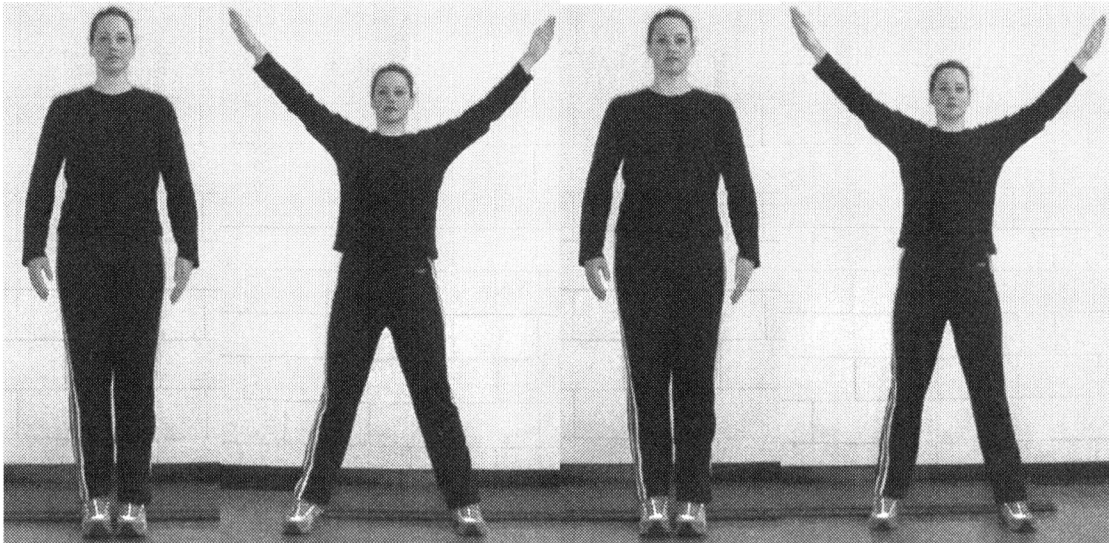

| Figure 1 | Figure 2 | Figure 3 | Figure 4 |

Muscles utilized: Shoulder, back, legs, butt.

Number of Repetitions: Goal 15-20, or if you are unable to complete the full 15-20 repetitions, attempt to complete 5 more repetitions beyond the point at which you begin to feel resistance.

Modified Jumping Jacks:

Figure 1. Start with feet together, standing comfortably.

Figure 2. Slide right leg outward to the side while simultaneously raising both hands.

Figure 3. Return to a relaxed state.

Figure 4. Slide left leg while simultaneously raising both hands.

Rest for a maximum of 2 minutes before starting the next exercise. As your fitness level improves decrease your rest time between each strength training exercise. We recommend that you decrease the rest time between each exercise by 15 seconds a week. The goal is to have 1 minute or less between exercises.

DAY 2. Exercise # 2: Chest Press

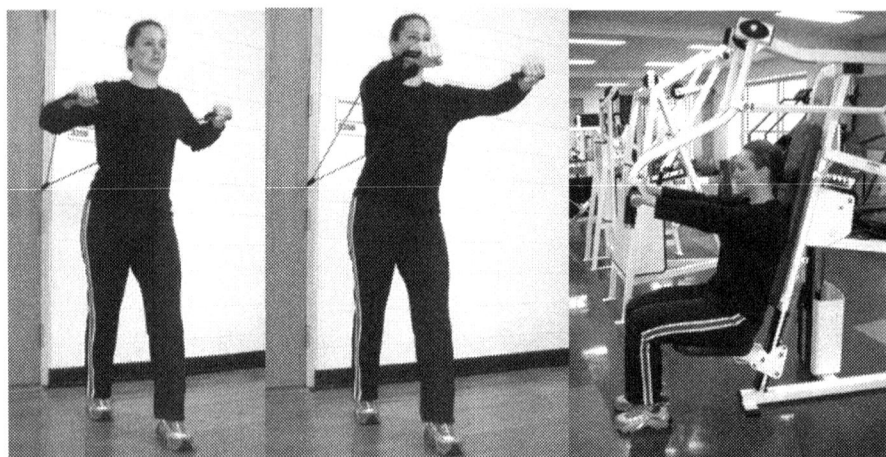

Figure 1   Figure 2   Figure 3

Muscles utilized: Chest (lower Pectoralis).

Number of Repetitions: Goal 15-20, or if you are unable to complete the full 15-20 repetitions, attempt to complete 5 more repetitions beyond the point at which you begin to feel resistance.

Figure1. (Start) Begin by feeding one end of the fitness tube through the loop of the door anchor until the loop is in the center of the fitness tube. The door anchor should be located at about shoulder height. Stand facing away from the fitness tube/anchor spot. Grasp the fitness tube handles and bring elbows up and out to each side.

Figure 2. (Finish) Standing with good, erect posture, push both arms straight out in front of the body, completely extending the elbows. Maintain arms at shoulder height throughout the exercise. Bring the elbows back to start position in a slow, controlled manner. Repeat 8-12 times.

Figure 3. Example of lower pectoralis press machine in a gym.

Rest for a maximum of 2 minutes before starting the next exercise. As your fitness level improves decrease your rest time between each strength training exercise. We recommend that you decrease the rest between each exercise by 15 seconds a week. The goal is to have 1 minute or less between exercises.

DAY 2. Exercise # 3: Chest Fly

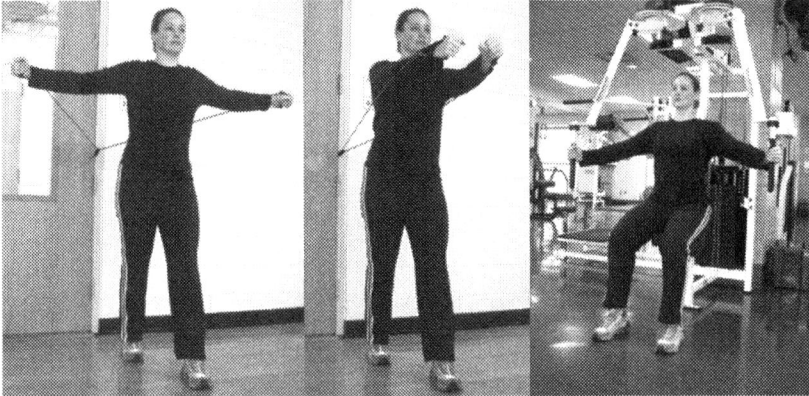

Figure 1   Figure 2   Figure 3

Muscles utilized: Chest (upper pectorals).

Number of Repetitions: Goal 15-20, or if you are unable to complete the full 15-20 repetitions, attempt to complete 5 more repetitions beyond the point at which you begin to feel resistance.

Figure1. (Start) Begin by feeding one end of the fitness tube through the loop of the door anchor until the loop is in the center of the fitness tube. The door anchor should be located at about shoulder height. Stand facing away from the anchor spot. Grasp the fitness tube handles and bring arms up and out to each side with a slight bend in the elbows.

Figure 2. (Finish) Standing with good, erect posture, push both arms straight out in front of the body, keeping the elbows locked. Maintain arms at shoulder height throughout the exercise. Bring the arms back to start position in a slow, controlled manner. Repeat 8-12 times.

Figure 3. Example of lower pectoralis press machine in a gym.

Rest for a maximum of 2 minutes before starting the next exercise. As your fitness level improves decrease your rest time between each strength training exercise. We recommend that you decrease the rest time between each exercise by 15 seconds a week. The goal is to have 1 minute or less between exercises.

DAY 2. Exercise #4: Modified Standing Row

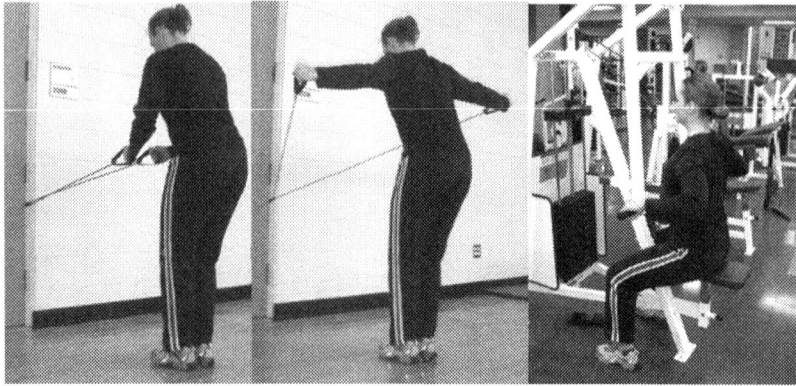

Figure 1   Figure 2   Figure 3

Muscles utilized: Upper and Mid-Back.

Number of Repetitions: Goal 15-20, or if you are unable to complete the full 15-20 repetitions, attempt to complete 5 more repetitions beyond the point at which you begin to feel resistance.

Figure1. (Start) Begin by feeding one end of the fitness tube through the loop of the door anchor until the loop is in the center of the fitness tube. The door anchor should be located at about mid-chest height. Facing the anchor point, grasp both fitness tube handles and extend your arms straight out in front of your body. Flex your torso to a 45 degree angle while maintaining a flat back.

Figure 2. (Finish) Pull both handles back toward your body, squeezing your shoulder blades together, until the elbows are bent and slightly behind your body in a standing position. Extend the arms back to the start position in a slow, controlled manner and repeat 8-12 times.

Figure 3. Example of a sitting row machine.

Rest for a maximum of 2 minutes before starting the next exercise. As your fitness level improves decrease your rest time between each strength training exercise. We recommend that you decrease the rest time between each exercise by 15 seconds a week. The goal is to have 1 minute or less between exercises.

DAY 2. Exercise #5: Cross Body Shoulder Rotation

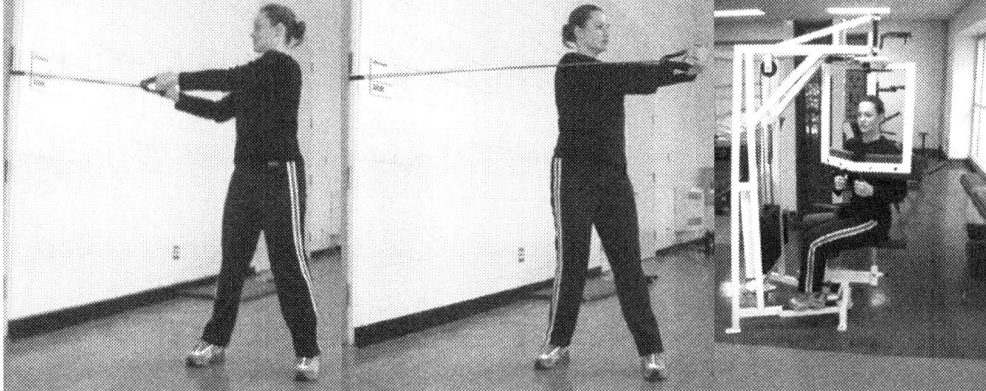

Figure 1   Figure 2   Figure 3

Muscles utilized: Chest, shoulders, latissimus dorsi.

Number of Repetitions: Goal 15-20, or if you are unable to complete the full 15-20 repetitions, attempt to complete 5 more repetitions beyond the point which you begin to feel resistance.

Figure1. (Start) Begin by feeding one end of the fitness tube through the loop of the door anchor until the loop is in the center of the fitness tube. The door anchor should be located at about shoulder height. Stand parallel from the anchor spot. Grasp the fitness tube handles and bring arms up and out to each side with a slight bend in the elbows.

Figure 2. (Finish) Standing with good, erect posture, push both arms straight out in front of the body, keeping the elbows locked. Maintain arms at shoulder height throughout the exercise, rotate your body slightly beyond the mid point. Bring the arms back to start position in a slow, controlled manner.

Figure 3. Example of torso rotation machine.

Rest for a maximum of 2 minutes before starting the next exercise. As your fitness level improves decrease your rest time between each strength training exercise. We recommend that you decrease the rest time between each exercise by 15 seconds a week. The goal is to have 1 minute or less between exercises.

DAY 2. Exercise #6: Full Body Extension

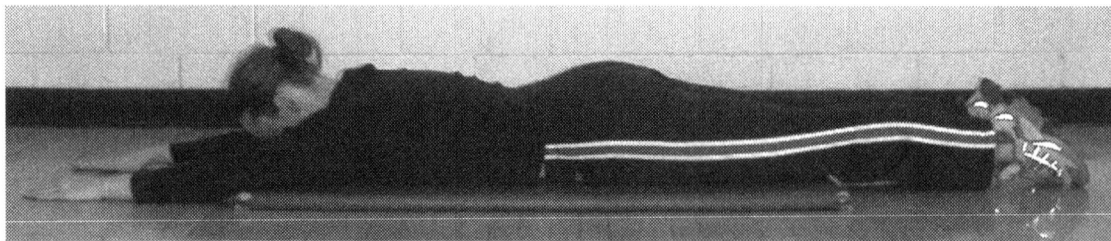
Figure 1

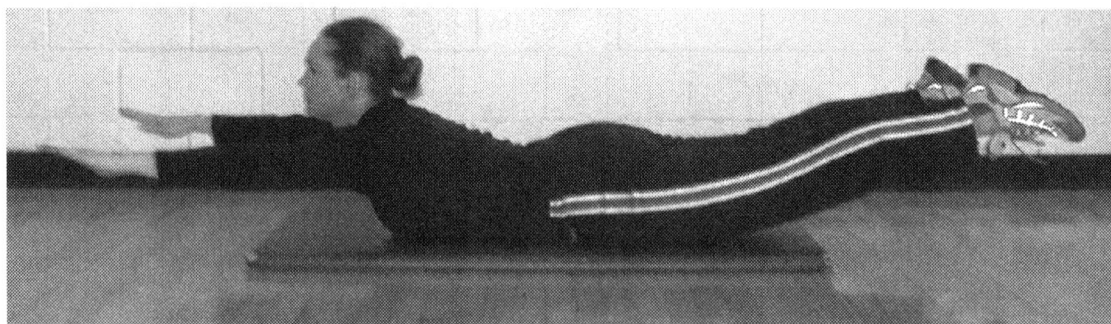
Figure 2

Muscles utilized: Lower back, abdominal, and buttocks.

Number of Repetitions: Goal 15-20, or if you are unable to complete the full 15-20 repetitions, attempt to complete 5 more repetitions beyond the point which you begin to feel resistance.

Figure 1. (Start) Lie on your stomach with extended arms and legs. Point your toes and keep your feet together.

Figure 2. (Finish) Lift your torso off the ground while simultaneously lifting legs off the floor. Hold position for 4-6 seconds. Return your legs to the starting position , relax, and repeat the exercise.

Rest for a maximum of 2 minutes before starting the next exercise. As your fitness level improves decrease your rest time between each strength training exercise. We recommend that you decrease the rest time between each exercise by 15 seconds a week. The goal is to have or 1 minute less between exercises.

DAY 2. Exercise #7: Modified Standing Row

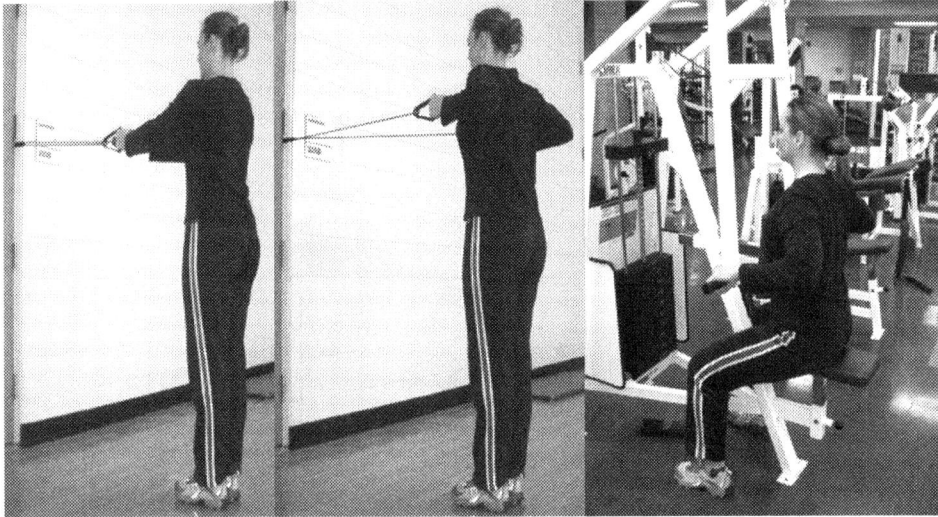

| Figure 1 | Figure 2 | Figure 3 |

Muscles utilized: Upper and mid back.

Number of Repetitions: Goal 15-20, or if you are unable to complete the full 15-20 repetitions, attempt to complete 5 more repetitions beyond the point which you begin to feel resistance.

Figure1. (Start) Begin by feeding one end of the fitness tube through the loop of the door anchor until the loop is in the center of the fitness tube. The door anchor should be located at about mid-chest height. Facing the anchor point, grasp both fitness tube handles and extend your arms straight out in front of your body.

Figure 2. (Finish) Pull both handles back toward your body, squeezing your shoulder blades together, until the elbows are bent and slightly behind your body in a standing position. Extend the arms back to the start position in a slow, controlled manner and repeat.

Figure 3. Example of a sitting row machine in a gym.

Rest for a maximum of 2 minutes before starting the next exercise. As your fitness level improves decrease your rest time between each strength training exercise. We recommend that you decrease the rest time between each exercise by 15 seconds a week. The goal is to have 1 minute or less between exercises.

DAY 2. Exercise #8: Lying Side Leg Raise

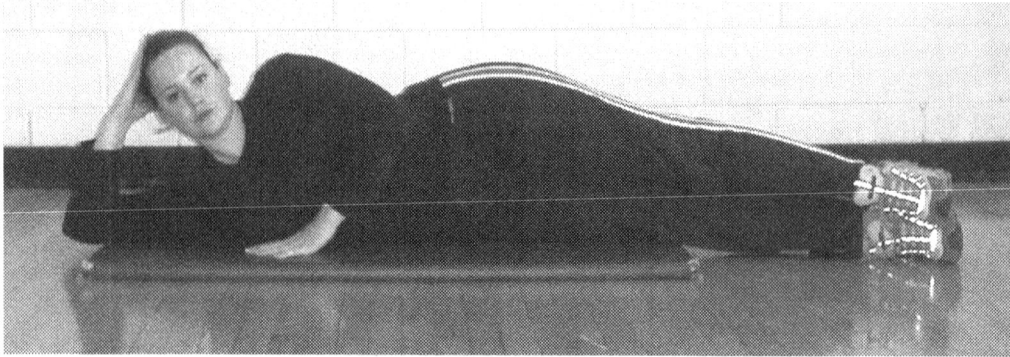

Figure 1

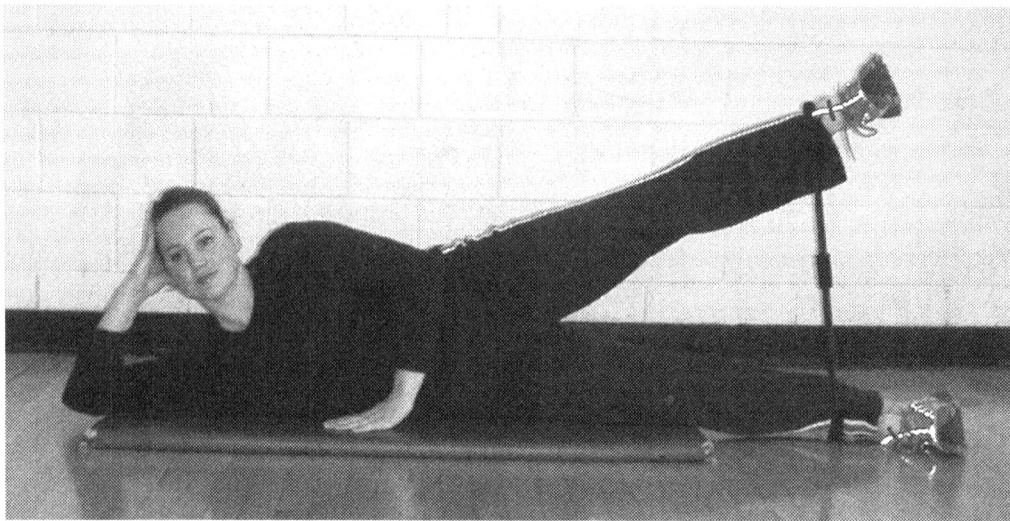

Figure 2

Muscles utilized: Groin, inner leg.

Number of Repetitions: Goal 15-20, or if you are unable to complete the full 15-20 repetitions, attempt to complete 5 more repetitions beyond the point at which you begin to feel resistance.

Figure 1. (Start) Place the figure-8 band around both ankles and lie on one side. Place one hand on the floor and support your head with the other hand as shown.

Lower figure. (Finish) With your hips square and upper body stationary, lift upper leg up and away from the side of your body to a comfortable height. Pause briefly and lower the leg slowly back to the start position. Repeat 15-20 times before turning to the opposite side to exercise the other leg.

Day 2 Exercise Review

Exercise # 1

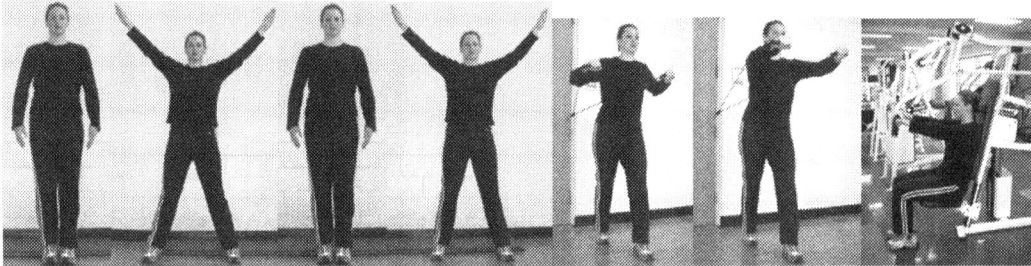

Fig 1   Fig 2   Fig 3   Fig 4

Exercise # 2

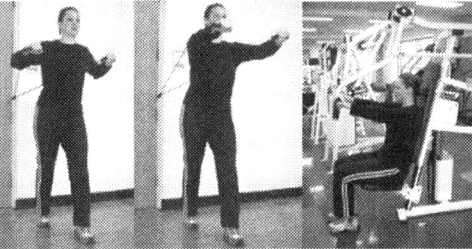

Fig 1   Fig 2   Fig 3

Exercise # 3

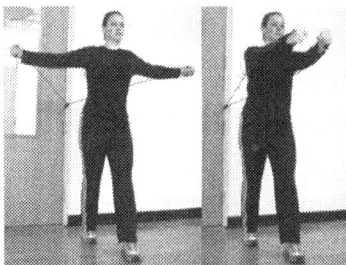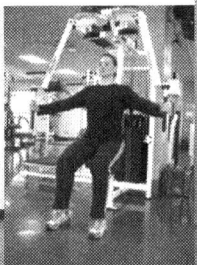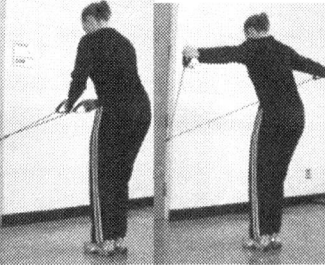

Fig 1   Fig 2   Fig 3

Exercise # 4

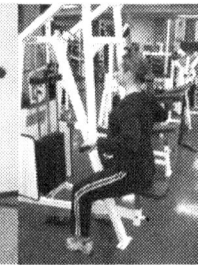

Fig 1   Fig 2   Fig 3

Exercise # 5

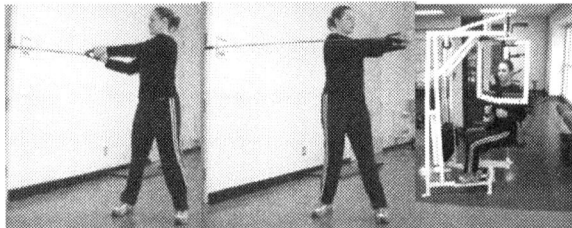

Fig 1   Fig 2   Fig 3

Exercise # 6

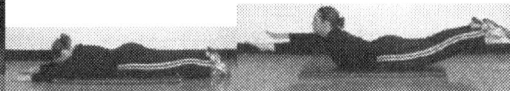

Fig 1   Fig 2

Exercise # 7

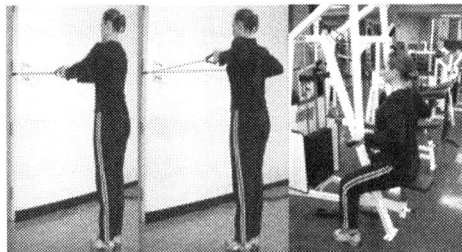

Fig 1   Fig 2   Fig 3

Exercise # 8

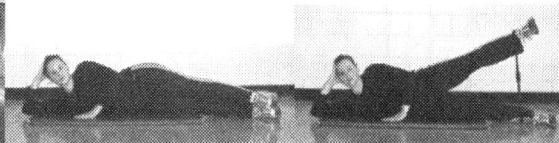

Fig 1   Fig 2

DAY 3. Exercise #1: Jumping Jacks Warm-Up

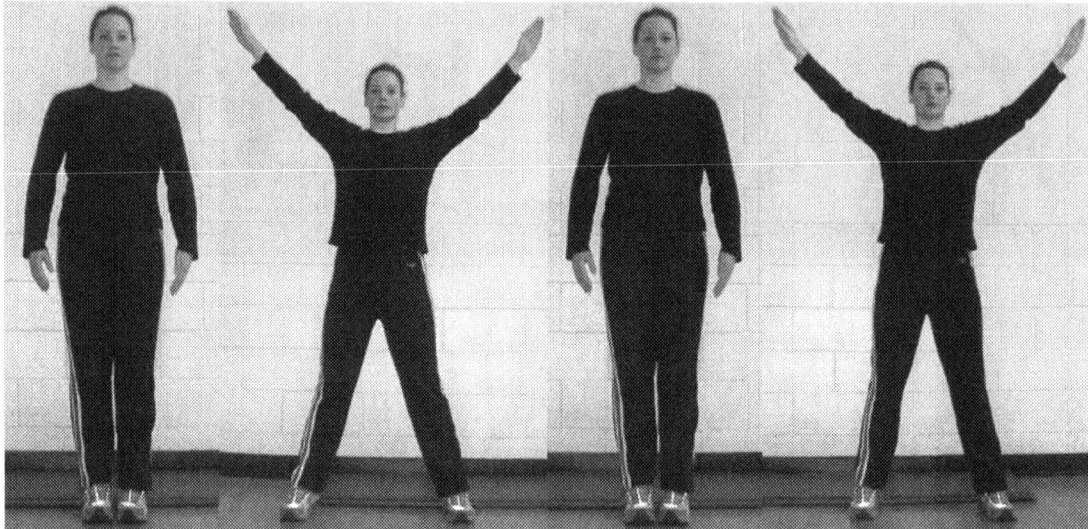

| Figure 1 | Figure 2 | Figure 3 | Figure 4 |

Muscles utilized: Shoulder, back, legs, butt.

Number of Repetitions: Goal 15-20, or if you are unable to complete the full 15-20 repetitions, attempt to complete 5 more repetitions beyond the point at which you begin to feel resistance.

Modified Jumping Jacks:

Figure 1. Start with legs together standing comfortably.

Figure 2. Slide right leg outward to the side while simultaneously raising both hands.

Figure 3. Return to a relaxed state.

Figure 4. Slide left leg while simultaneously raising both hands.

Rest for a maximum of 2 minutes before starting the next exercise. As your fitness level improves decrease your rest time between each strength training exercise. We recommend that you decrease the rest time between each exercise by 15 seconds a week. The goal is to have 1 minute or less between exercises.

DAY 3. Exercise #2: Triceps Extension

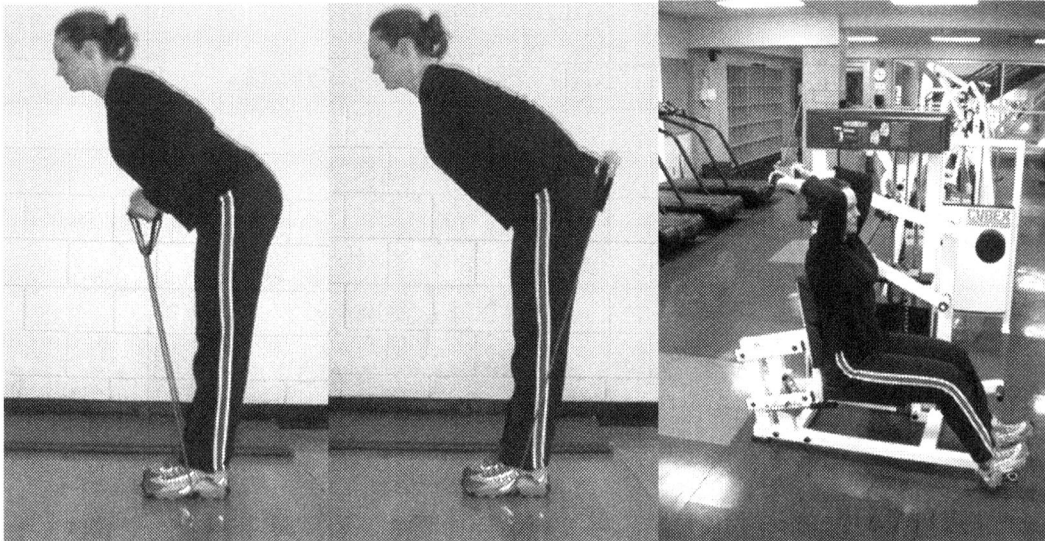

Figure 1   Figure 2   Figure 3

Muscles utilized: Triceps.

Number of Repetitions: Goal 15-20, or if you are unable to complete the full 15-20 repetitions, attempt to complete 5 more repetitions beyond the point at which you begin to feel resistance.

Figure 1. (Start) Place resistance cord firmly under your feet. Grasp resistance cord handles, keep arms close to your body. Stand up. Bend your torso forward to achieve a 45 degree angle, keep your back flat, and look forward.

Figure 2. (Finish) Push your hands back until your arms are extended. Pause, then slowly recover to the starting position.

Figure 3. Example of a triceps extension machine.

Rest for a maximum of 2 minutes before starting the next exercise. As your fitness level improves decrease your rest time between each strength training exercise. We recommend that you decrease the rest time between each exercise by 15 seconds a week. The goal is to have 1 minute or less between exercises.

DAY 3. Exercise #3: Body Arch

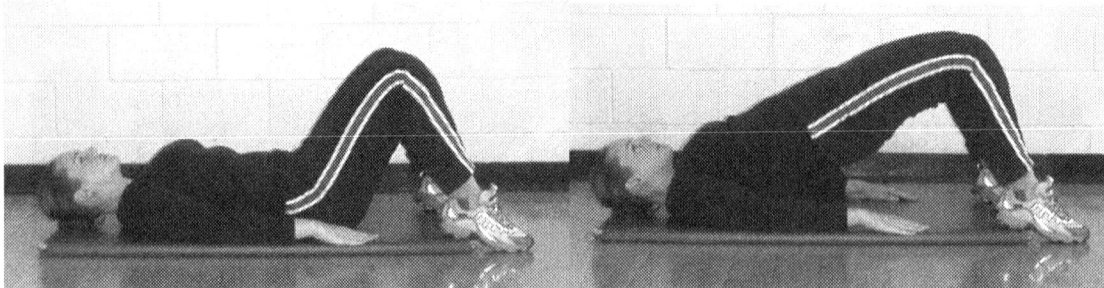

Figure 1   Figure 2

Muscles utilized: Legs, buttocks, stomach.

Number of Repetitions: Goal 15-20, or if you are unable to complete the full 15-20 repetitions, attempt to complete 5 more repetitions beyond the point at which you begin to feel resistance.

Figure 1. (Start) Lie on floor, with feet firmly placed on the floor, knees bent, arms at sides.

Figure 2. (Finish) Raise buttocks off floor while keeping your feet firmly placed on the floor, and shoulders firmly placed on the floor.

Rest for a maximum of 2 minutes before starting the next exercise. As your fitness level improves decrease your rest time between each strength training exercise. We recommend that you decrease the rest time between each exercise by 15 seconds a week. The goal is to have 1 minute or less between exercises.

DAY 3. Exercise #4: Trunk Twisting Sit-Up

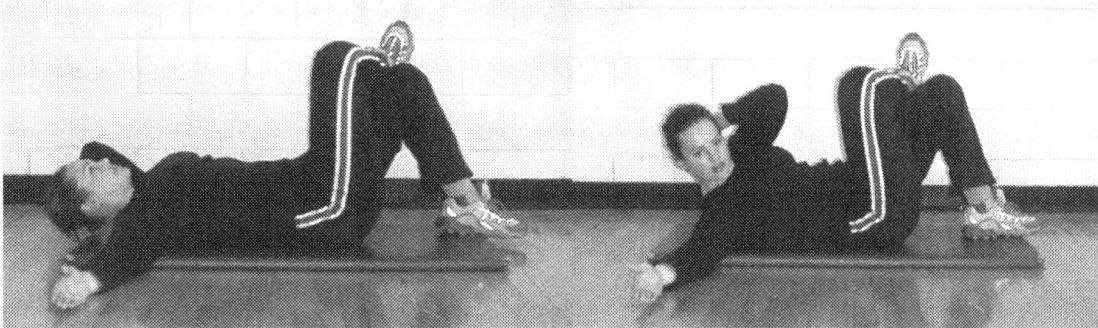

Figure 1   Figure 2

Muscles utilized: Stomach, obliques.

Number of Repetitions: Goal 15-20, or if you are unable to complete the full 15-20 repetitions, attempt to complete 5 more repetitions beyond the point at which you begin to feel resistance.

Figure1. (Start) Lie with your knees bent, one leg crossed over the other leg, and your one hand behind your head, and your other hand outstretched for stability.

Figure 2. (Finish) Turn to your left as far as possible, and extend your elbow towards your opposing knee. Quickly turn to your right, and repeat the motion. Repeat in succession to the left, right.

Rest for a maximum of 2 minutes before starting the next exercise. As your fitness level improves decrease your rest time between each strength training exercise. We recommend that you decrease the rest time between each exercise by 15 seconds a week. The goal is to have 1 minute or less between exercises.

DAY 3. Exercise #5. Push-Up with Knee Support (upper pictures)/Push-Up Without Knee Support (lower pictures)

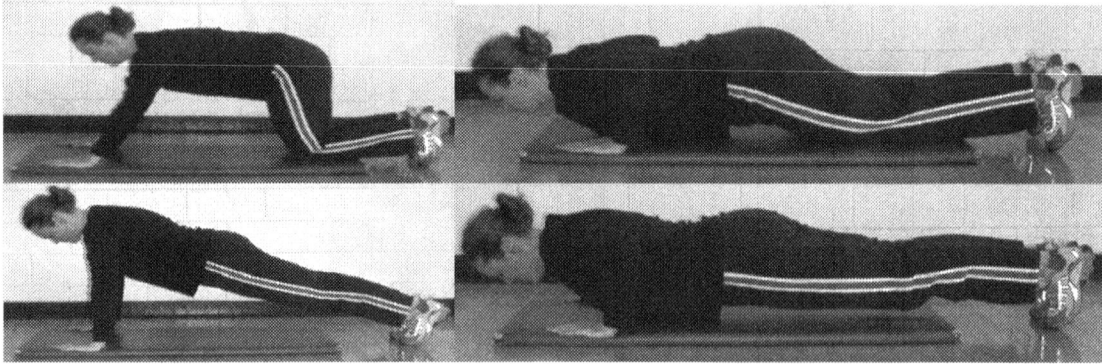

Figure 1   Figure 2

Muscles utilized: Pectoralis, shoulder, deltoid.

Number of Repetitions: Goal 15-20, or if you are unable to complete the full 15-20 repetitions, attempt to complete 5 more repetitions beyond the point at which you begin to feel resistance.

Figure 1. (Start, upper photo) With your body supported on your extended arms and knees.

Figure 1. (Start, lower photo) With your body supported on your extended arms and feet.

Figure 2. (Finish, upper and lower photo) Slowly lower your chest to the floor by bending your elbows. Keep your back straight and your head up; don't let your hips or thighs touch the floor while you are doing push-ups. Repeat in succession, barely touching your chest to the floor with each push-up.

Rest for a maximum of 2 minutes before starting the next exercise. As your fitness level improves decrease your rest time between each strength training exercise. We recommend that you decrease the rest time between each exercise by 15 seconds a week. The goal is to have 1 minute or less between exercises.

DAY # 3. Exercise #6: Forward Lunge

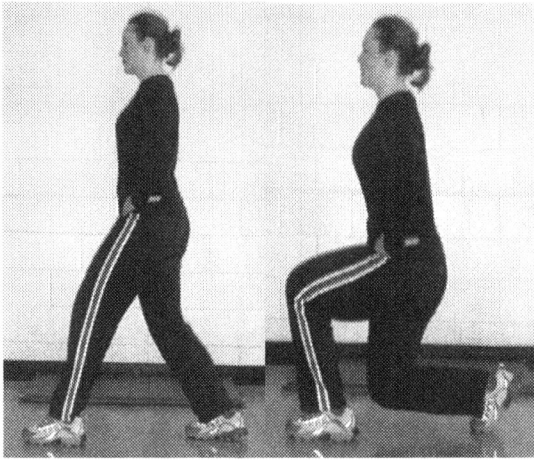

Figure 1   Figure 2

If you have a history of knee problems/knee ligament injuries, you may skip this exercise as it does produce a significant amount of strain on your knees.

Muscles utilized: Quadriceps, buttocks, hamstrings.

Number of Repetitions: Goal 15-20, or if you are unable to complete the full 15-20 repetitions, attempt to complete 5 more repetitions beyond the point at which you begin to feel resistance.

Figure 1. (Start) Stand with your arms at your sides, hands on hips. Your feet should be comfortably together, and your head should remain erect.

Figure 2. (Finish) Stride forward with one leg. Slowly lower your body so that your upper (front) leg is parallel to the ground and your rear leg is slightly extended. Your back knee should gently touch the floor. Push back with your front leg, keeping your trunk erect. Pause, then slowly recover to the starting position. Alternate legs. Try to push back with enough force to prevent your front heel from dragging on the floor.

Rest for a maximum of 2 minutes before starting the next exercise. As your fitness level improves decrease your rest time between each strength training exercise. We recommend that you decrease the rest time between each exercise by 15 seconds a week. The goal is to have less than 1 minute between exercises.

DAY #3. Exercise #7: Flutter Kick

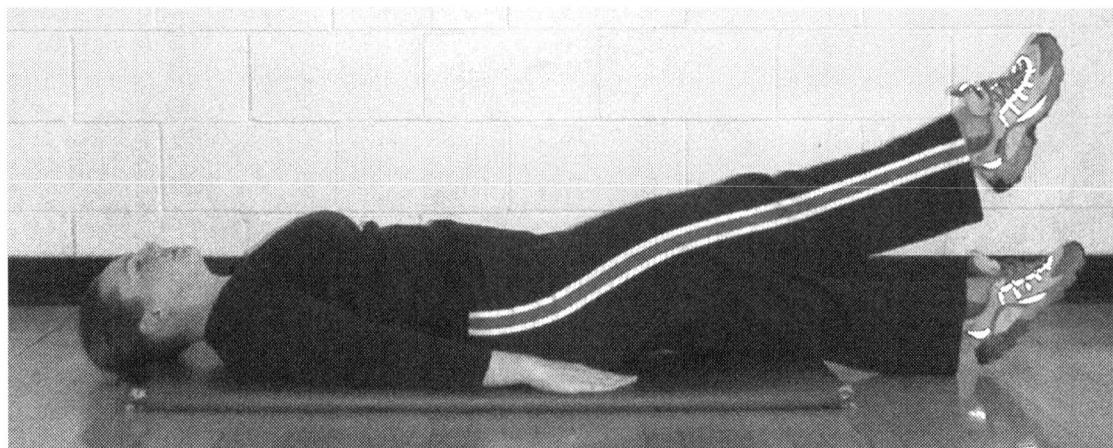

Muscles utilized: Abdominals.

Number of Repetitions: Goal 15-20, or if you are unable to complete the full 15-20 repetitions, attempt to complete 5 more repetitions beyond the point at which you begin to feel resistance.

Figure 1. Lie on your back, with your hands at your side and your feet on the floor. Point your toes, lift both legs up off the floor and flutter kick for five seconds. Return your legs to the starting position. Relax for 10-30 seconds then repeat the kick.

Rest for a maximum of 2 minutes before starting the next exercise. As your fitness level improves decrease your rest time between each strength training exercise. We recommend that you decrease the rest time between each exercise by 15 seconds a week. The goal is to have 1 minute or less between exercises.

DAY #3. Exercise #8: Step-Up

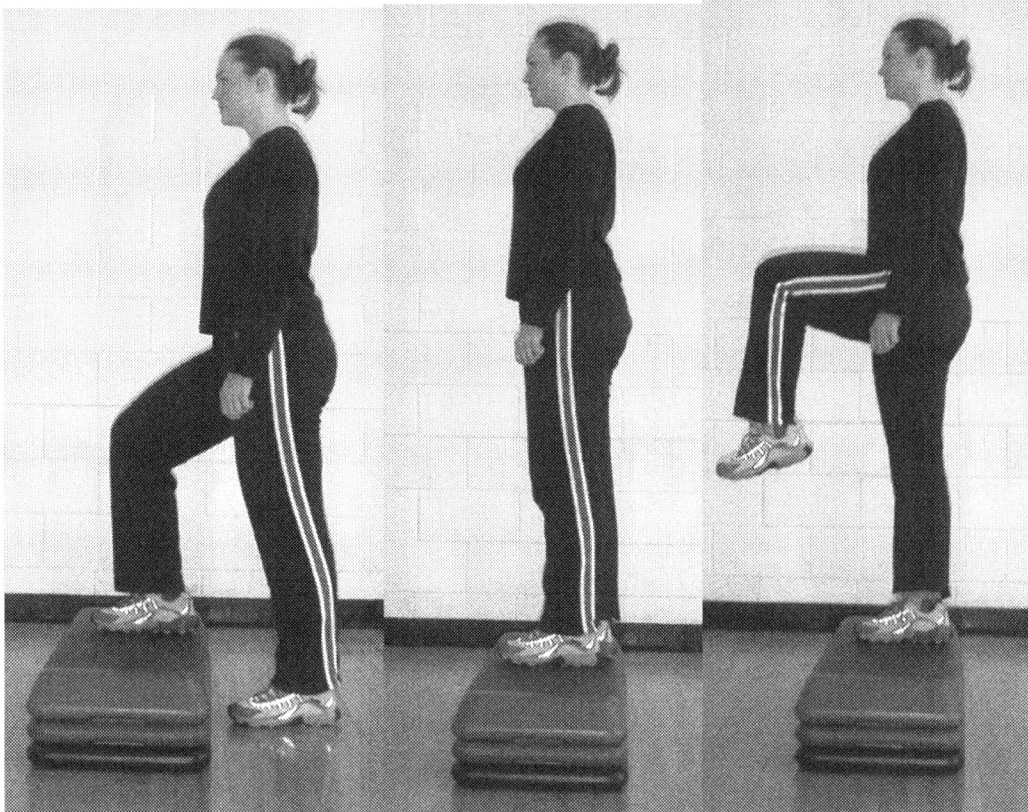

Figure 1   Figure 2   Figure 3

Muscles utilized: Quadriceps, buttocks, hip flexors.

Number of Repetitions: Goal 15-20, or if you are unable to complete the full 15-20 repetitions, attempt to complete 5 more repetitions beyond the point at which you begin to feel resistance.

Figure 1. Beginning with left leg, step up onto a bench or block, and lift your body with that leg.

Figure 2. Stand on bench with both feet.

Figure 3. Drive the knee of your right leg up. Step down from the bench, and alternate lead legs.

Day 3 Exercise Review

Exercise # 1

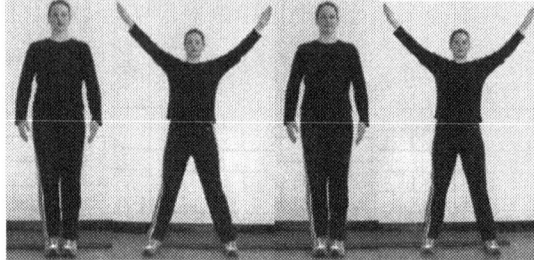

Fig 1 Fig 2 Fig 3 Fig 4

Exercise # 2

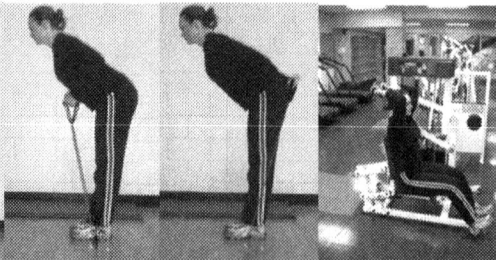

Fig 1 Fig 2 Fig 3

Exercise # 3

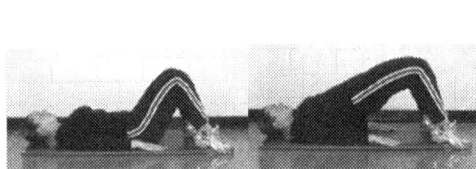

Fig 1 Fig 2

Exercise # 4

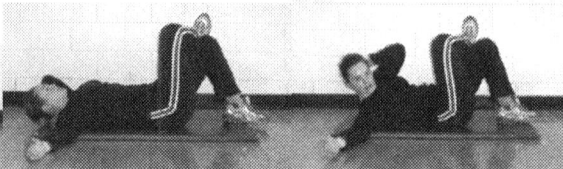

Fig 1 Fig 2

Exercise # 5

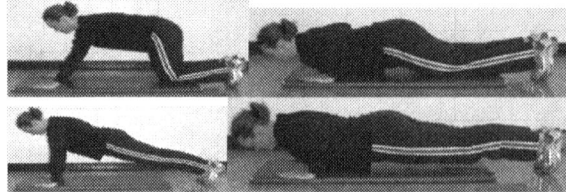

Fig 1 Fig 2

Exercise # 6

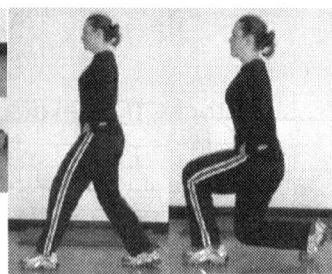

Fig 1 Fig 2

Exercise # 7

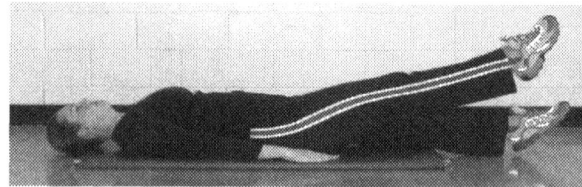

Exercise # 8

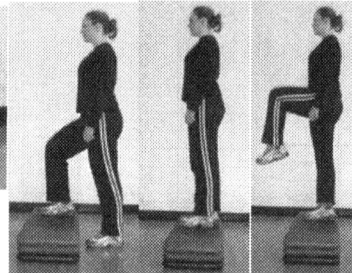

Fig1 Fig 2 Fig 3

Alternate Exercise Regimen

Some individuals may find the exercise goals listed and explained in Part Six to be intimidating. If you are a person who wants to begin an exercise plan, but at a slower pace, the following regimen may be more suitable to your current level of conditioning.

1) Complete 10 minutes of moderate daily activity. Moderate activity is activity which can be completed while comfortably talking to another individual. Examples of potential activities are: a brisk walk, riding a stationary bike or regular bike (weather permitting), a light run, swim or water aerobics.

2) Increase daily activity level by 10 minutes each month for six months. By the end of six months you should be completing 60 minutes of moderate activity each day. Sixty minutes of moderate activity is also the equivalent of 10,000 steps a day on a pedometer. A pedometer is an inexpensive device which can be purchased at any sporting goods store or department store. It is worn on your waistband and it measures the number of steps, or up and down movements an individual completes.

3) Once you have achieved 60 minutes of daily activity you may choose to continue to complete 60 minutes of moderate activity or intensify your efforts toward reaching the equivalent of 30 minutes of strenuous activity on a daily basis. Strenuous activity is activity in which an individual could not comfortably carry on a

conversation with another individual. An example of strenuous activity is a light jog. Remember, moderate or strenuous activity can be completed in 10-minute blocks if desired. Your ultimate goal is to achieve either 60 minutes of moderate or 30 minutes of vigorous activity on a daily basis.

Graphical Representation of Alternate Exercise Goals

Month 1	Month 2	Month 3	Month 4	Month 5	Month 6
10 min of moderate daily actvity	20 min of moderate daily actvity	30 min of moderate daily actvity	40 min of moderate daily actvity	50 min of moderate daily actvity	60 min of moderate daily actvity
			or	or	or
			20 min of vigorous daily actvity	25min of vigorous daily actvity	30 min of vigorous daily actvity

Continue month 6 activity levels to maintain a stable weight.

Part Seven:
Key Components of a Healthy Lifestyle

Adequate Sleep
Daily Vitamins/Supplements
Stress Reduction
Limit Fast Food Consumption

A healthy lifestyle is dependent upon many factors. Maintenance of a stable appropriate weight is very important. In order, to achieve maximal health benefits you must also make efforts to change other aspects of your life.

Adequate Sleep

Appropriate levels of sleep are required for health. I recommend obtaining 7 hours of sleep a night. A large scale study conducted by Dr. Daniel Kripe at the University of California revealed that people who slept seven hours per night had the lowest death rates over a six-year period, while people who slept eight or more hours had a greater risk of dying over the same period. The greater the sleep duration beyond eight hours per night, the greater the death rate and people who slept five hours per night lived longer than those who slept eight or more. Therefore, too little or too much sleep can be unhealthy, but optimal sleep time of 7 hours, may help you to live longer.

Daily Vitamins/Supplements

I recommend for all adults, over 18 years old, daily:

> A multivitamin
> Calcium Carbonate, 1200 mg
> Vitamin D, a total of 1000 I.U.
> Fish Oil, 1000-3000 mg

<u>Multivitamin</u>: It is essential to achieve adequate levels of vitamins and minerals on a daily basis. Vitamin and mineral supplements should not be taken as a substitute for a healthy and nutritious diet. However, very few individuals consume the recommended minimum five servings of fruit and vegetables on a given day. Therefore, I recommend that all individuals, eighteen years of age and up, supplement their diet with a daily multivitamin. Any weight-loss program should encourage the consumption of a daily multivitamin. A multicenter study in 2001 revealed significantly decreased levels of vitamin E, calcium, iron, and zinc during the first four months of a weight-loss program. The authors concluded that during the initial phase of such a regimen, a multivitamin supplement should be considered to ensure adequate intake of Vitamin E, zinc, calcium and folate.

<u>Calcium</u>: The preferred source of calcium is through calcium-rich foods such as dairy products. Each serving of dairy (8 oz glass of milk, slice of cheese, or 2 cups of 1% or 2% cottage cheese) contains approximately 300 mg of calcium. Unfortunately, consuming 3-4 servings of dairy food on a daily basis is very difficult to integrate into a lower-calorie diet. Therefore I recommend that all individuals supplement with

1000 mg of calcium carbonate in the form of tablets or chews on a daily basis. The optimal calcium intake for most individuals is greater than 1000 mg a day and can be achieved with additional dietary calcium intake. Calcium intake up to a total of 2000 mg a day appears to be safe in most individuals.

Optimal Calcium Intake

Young adults, 11-24 years of age	1000 mg a day
Women, 25-50 years of age	1200-1500 mg a day
Lactating or pregnant women	1200-1500 mg a day
Postmenopausal women on estrogen replacement	1000 mg a day
Postmenopausal women not on estrogen replacement	1500 mg a day
Males 25-65 years of age	1000 mg a day
Menopausal women, greater then 65 years of age	1500 mg a day

Vitamin D: I strongly recommend the consumption of 1000 International Units of Vitamin D a day. Vitamin D can easily be consumed in tablet form. Milk in the United States is fortified with 400 International Units (I.U.) of Vitamin D per quart. However, very few individuals consume enough milk products on a daily basis to achieve 1000 I.U.

Benefits of Vitamin D include:
* Vitamin D reduces the risk of colon cancer.
* Clinical studies have shown Vitamin D deficiencies to be associated with four of the most common cancers, breast, prostate, colon, and skin.
* Vitamin D aids in the absorption of calcium, helping to form and maintain strong bones.
* Vitamin D deficiency has been associated with insulin deficiency and insulin resistance. Insulin resistance

promotes heart disease, the number one cause of death and disability in the United States.

* Progression of degenerative arthritis of the knee and hip is faster in people with lower Vitamin D concentrations.

<u>Fish Oil</u>: Current recommendations for fish oil are 1000-3000 mg a day. A growing body of evidence suggests individuals can reduce their risk of developing heart disease, cancer, and Alzheimer's by consuming a diet high in Omega-3 fatty acids. Omega-3 fatty acids are found in oily fish such as salmon, flounder and cod. Fish oil supplements are also a good source of Omega-3 fatty acids. Oily fish should be, at a minimum, consumed once a week. However, most health experts agree that certain individuals, particularly pregnant women and young children, should avoid fish known to be contaminated with high levels of methyl-mercury. These fish include sword fish, shark, and Albacore tuna.

Stress Reduction

Reduction of stress is essential for a healthy and productive life. Stress is inevitable, however too much stress can lead to heart disease, high blood pressure, and cancer, and may be connected to other conditions: asthma, allergies, migraines, ulcers, bowel and skin problems. I strongly recommend daily activity as a measure for reducing stress levels. My personal favorite is a mixture of strength training and aerobic exercise (see Part Six). However, many other valid and effective forms of stress relief are effective, including yoga, Pilates, meditation, and martial arts. Other techniques which can assist in reducing daily stress are the following:

* Rise early, set aside time to organize the day.
* Share your workload with others, coworkers and family members.
* Learn to say no.
* Set reasonable goals.
* Practice patience.
* Always set time aside to exercise.
* Learn from your mistakes and attempt to not repeat the behaviors or associated actions.

Limit Fast Food Consumption

Fast food consumption is strongly associated with weight gain and insulin resistance. A recent study completed at the University of Minnesota found that individuals who frequented fast food restaurants more often over a 15 year period gained more weight and developed insulin resistance. Insulin resistance increases an individual's chances of developing diabetes. The development of diabetes is associated with many health risks if not effectively managed, including damage to an individual's eyes, heart, kidneys and nervous system.

Here are some simple tips to eat more healthfully at restaurants.
* Try to consume foods that are baked, grilled, dry-sautéed, broiled, poached, or steamed. These cooking techniques utilize less fat.
* Choose entrees with fruits and vegetables as key ingredients.

* Choose foods made with whole grains, such as whole-wheat bread, brown rice, or wild rice.
* Ask the server to substitute vegetables or a baked potato for French fries.
* Order salad dressings on the side and use less.
* Choose salad dressings that are 'light' or low-fat.
* If pasta dishes are ordered, choose tomato-basil sauces rather then cream-based sauces.
* Share appetizers and desserts with a friend.
* If the food cannot be shared, bring half of your meal home.
* Drink water, diet soda (pop), or unsweetened tea in place of regular soda (pop) or alcoholic beverages.
* Do not deprive yourself of the foods you love. Eat them in smaller quantities and/or share with friends.

Part Eight: Personalizing the North Star Diet Program and Questions Answered

Why am I not achieving my weight-loss goals utilizing the North Star Diet and Weight Maintenance Program?

You may not achieve your weight-loss goals following the North Star Diet and Weight Management Program in two circumstances:

1) An individual does not comply with the calorie-restrictive diets (Part Three and Four).

In order to make sure that you are complying with the diet requirements it is a good practice to keep a log of everything you eat in a day. This is a proven technique used by successful dieters. See the appendix for a sample calorie log.

2) There is the rare possibility that your calculated REE (resting energy expenditure) is 1200 or fewer calories.

This second possibility is somewhat more complicated. Resting energy expenditure is equal to the number of calories required to maintain weight. All weight loss is dependent on one simple fact. To lose weight individuals must consume fewer calories than their calculated REE. REE can be calculated by using the Revised Harris-Benedict Equation. The Revised Harris-Benedict Equation takes into account an individual's gender, height, weight and age. The REE can be calculated by inputting your height, weight and age in the appropriate equation. If you have access to the internet you may calculate your REE, quickly at the following website:

http://wwwusers.med.cornell.edu/~spon/picu/calc/beecalc.htm

Revised Harris-Benedict Equation

MALES
66.5 +(6.25 x lbs) +(12.7 x inches) – (6.77 x Age) =REE

FEMALES
665.1 +(4.34x lb) + (4.7 x inches) – (4.676 x Age) =REE

REE is expressed in calories per day.
Height is expressed in inches.
Weight is expressed in pounds.
Age is expressed in years.

To lose weight individuals must decrease their caloric intake by multiplying their calculated REE x .8. Again, in order to lose weight your caloric intake must be lower than your REE. Therefore, if your calculated REE is 1200, you will not lose weight if you consume 1200 calories. Weight loss will only occur if the caloric intake is decreased by 250 calories, or 1200 calories x .8. The North Star Diet and Weight Management System purposely does not contain a sub-1200 calorie diet as it often produces malnutrition in individuals unless followed precisely. We strongly recommend that if your calculated REE x .8 is less than 1200 calories that you meet with a nutritionist or physician comfortable with weight-loss management to help you construct a safe caloric diet of fewer than 1200 calories.

How do you determine your weight maintenance caloric requirements?

Once you have achieved your weight-loss goals, efforts should be directed at maintaining your desired weight. The North Star Diet and Weight Maintenance Program is greatly concerned with individuals achieving weight loss and maintaining their desired weight. The maintenance of a stable, non-fluctuating weight is dependent on two factors, 60-90 minutes of moderate daily exercise and accurate determination of the Resting Energy Expenditure (REE). Resting Energy Expenditure is the amount of daily energy, in calories, required to maintain an individual's weight. REE can be calculated by utilizing the Revised Harris-Benedict Equation described in the previous discussion. You will now use your REE to find your weight-maintenance calorie requirements by multiplying that number by a coefficient which may be anywhere from 1.0 to 2.0.

Once you have calculated your REE, I recommend that you start by multiplying the REE value by 1.2. Consume the calculated daily amount of calories for a week. If your weight decreases during that week you must adjust your intake upward. Multiply by 1.3 or 1.4, increasing your caloric consumption accordingly until your weight remains stable. The coefficient by which you multiply the REE will vary in individuals depending on the amount of exercise done on a daily basis, muscle mass, and the amount of fidgeting they do. Therefore, individuals who exercise more daily, have a greater muscle mass, or have a higher metabolism will have proportionally greater caloric requirements. Once you have accurately determined your individual REE, attempt to consume the designated caloric amount to maintain your weight loss.

Are prescription weight-loss medications safe and effective?

At this time I do not recommend the use of weight-loss medications. Three preparations are currently licensed in the United States: Phetermine, Orlistat, and Meridia. Each produces weight loss in obese patients. However, the weight loss is modest, and in most cases the lost weight is regained when treatment is stopped. Health benefits can only be achieved with a sustained reduction in weight, and it seems likely that drug treatments would have to be taken indefinitely for weight loss to be sustained. Currently, there is little data on either the long-term safety or improvement of health for either Meridia or Orlistat. Phentermine is only approved for short term use, such as a few weeks. It should not be used by people with heart disease, high blood pressure, or an overactive thyroid gland. The medication is associated with a signifcant potential for physical dependence or addiction.

Does weight-loss surgery cure obesity?

Bariatric surgery, also commonly known as weight-loss surgery, is currently the most successful approach to treating obesity and reversing or preventing the development of several diseases associated with obesity. However, it is not a cure. Between 25-30% of individuals who have bariatric surgery in the United States will have regained all of their weight by five years following the procedure. The failure rate is associated with the inability to make lifestyle changes, most importantly daily exercise and maintaining appropriate caloric intake. All individuals who have bariatric surgery will rapidly lose significant weight in the one to one and a half years following surgery. Unfortunately, if lifestyle changes are not incorporated following this rapid weight loss, individuals will gain weight, and approximately one quarter to one third of all patients will regain all of their previous weight.

Part Nine:
Helpful Program Aids and Resources

Fiber chart

Resting energy equations

Caloric diary sample page

Exercise diary sample pages

North Star Diet rules

Exercise review: Days 1-3

Fiber Chart

Food	Portion	Calories	Fiber (grams)
Almonds:			
Slivered	1 tbsp	14	0.6
Sliced	1/4 cup	56	2.4
Apple:			
Raw	1 small	55-60	3.0
Raw	1 medium	70	4.0
Raw	1 large	80-100	4.5
Baked	1 large	100	5.0
Applesauce:	2/3 cup	182	3.6
Apricots:			
Raw	1 half	17	0.8
Dried	2 halves	36	1.7
Canned In syrup	3 halves	86	2.5
Artichokes:			
Cooked	1 large	30-44	4.5
Canned Hearts	4 or 4 small	24	4.5
Asparagus:			
Cooked, small spears	1/2 cup	17	1.7
Avocado:			
Diced	1/4 cup	97	1.7
Sliced	2 slices	50	0.9
Whole	1/2 avg.. size	170	2.8
Bacon: Flavored chips (imitation)	1 tbsp.	32	0.7
Baked beans:			
in sauce (8-oz can)	1 cup	180	16.0
with pork & molasses	1 cup	200-260	16.0
Baked potato: (see potatoes)			
Banana: Raw	1 medium 8"	96	3.0
Beans:			
Black, cooked	1 cup	190	19.4
Broad beans (Italian, haricot)	3/4 cup	30	3.0
Great Northern Kidney beans	1 cup	160	16.0
Lima beans	1/2 cup	118	3.7
Lima, dried, canned or cooked	1/2 cup	150	5.8
Pinto, dried before cooking	1/2 cup	155	18.8
Pinto, canned or cooked	1 cup	155	18.8
White, dried before cooking	1/2 cup	160	16.0
Canned or cooked	1/2 cup	160	16.0
(See also Green (snap) beans,			
(Chickpeas, Peas, Lentils)			
Bean sprouts: Raw in salad	1/4 cup	7	0.8
Beet greens: Cooked (see Greens)			
Beets:			
Cooked, sliced	1/2 cup	33	2.5
Whole	3 small	48	3.7
Blackberries:			
Raw, no sugar	1/2 cup	27	4.4
Canned, in juice	1/2 cup	54	5.0
Jam, with seeds	1 tbsp.	60	0.7
Bran Meal:	3 tbsp	28	6.0
Bran muffins: (see muffins)			
Brazil nuts: Shelled	2	48	2.5

Food	Portion	Calories	Fiber (grams)
Bread:			
Boston Brown cracked	2 slices	100	4.0
Wheat	2 slices	120	3.6
(Natural Ovens Bakery) Wheat high-bran bread	2 slices	120-160	8.0
White	2 slices	160	1.9
Rye (whole grain)	2 slices	160	1.9
Pumpernickel	2 slices	116	4.0
Seven-grain	2 slices	111-140	6.5
Whole Wheat	2 slices	120	6.0
Whole Wheat raisin	2 slices	120	6.0
Bread crumbs, whole wheat	1 tbsp	22	2.5
Broccoli:			
Raw	1/2 cup	20	4.0
Frozen	4 spears	20	5.0
Fresh, cooked	3/4 cup	30.0	7.0
Brussel sprouts cooked:	3/4 cup	36	3.0
Buckwheat groats:			
(kasha) before cooking	1/2 cup	160	9.6
Cooked	1 cup	160	9.6
Bulgur: soaked and cooked	1 cup	160	9.6
Cabbage: White or red			
Raw	1/2 cup	8	1.5
Cooke	2/3 cup	15	3.0
Cantaloupe: Raw	1/4	38	1.0
Carrots:			
Raw, (4-5 sticks)	1/4 cup	10	1.7
Cooked	1/2 cup	20	3.4
Catsup: see tomatoes			
Cauliflower:			
Raw, chopped	3 tiny buds	10	1.2
Cooked, chopped	7/8 cup	16	2.3
Celery:			
Raw	1/4 cup	5	2.0
Chopped	2 tbsp	3	1.0
Cooked	1/2 cup	9	3.0
Cereal:			
All-Bran	3 tbsp	35	5.0
Bran Buds	1/2 cup	90	10.4
	3 tbsp	35	5.0
	1/2 cup	90	10.0
Bran Chex	2/3 cup	90	5.0
Bran Flakes, Plain	1 cup	90	5.0
Bran Flakes, with raisins	1 cup	90	6.0
Corn flakes	3/4 cup	70	206
Cracklin' Brand	1/2 cup	110	4.0
Most bran cereals	1 cup	200	8.0
Oatmeal	3/4 cup	212	4.0
Puffed wheat	1 cup	43	3.3
Raisin Bran	1 cup	195	5.0
Wheatena	2/3 cup	101	2.2
Wheaties	1 cup	104	2.0
Cherries: Sweet, raw	10	28	1.2
	1/2 cup	55	1.0
Chestnuts roasted:	2 large	29	1.9
Chickpeas (garbanzos):			
Canned	1/2 cup	86	6.0
Cooked	1 cup	172	12.0
Coconut:			
Dried sweetened	1 tbsp	46	3.4
Unsweetened	1 tbsp	22	3.4
Corn:			
(Sweet) on cob	1 medium ear	64-70	5.0
Kernels, cooked or canned	1/2 cup	64	5.0
Cream-style, canned	1/2 cup	64	5.0
Succotash (with limas)	1/2 cup	66	7.0
Cornbread:	1 sq. (2 1/2")	93	3.4

Food	Portion	Calories	Fiber (grams)
Crackers:			
Cream	2	50	0.4
Graham	2	53	1.4
Ry-Krisp	3	64	2.3
Triscuits	2	50	2.0
Wheat Thins	6	58	2.2
Cranberries:			
Raw	1/4 cup	12	2.0
Sauce	1/2 cup	45	4.0
Cranberry-orange relish	1 tbsp	56	0.5
Cucumber: Raw unpeeled	10 thin slices	12	0.7
Dates: Pitted	2 (1/2 oz.)	39	1.2
Eggplant: Baked with Tomatoes	2 thick slices	42	4.0
Endive: Raw	10 leaves	10	0.6
English muffins: (see muffins)			
Figs:			
Dried	3	120	10.5
Fresh	1	30	2.0
Fruit N' Fiber Cereal:	1/2 cup	90	3.5
Graham Crackers: (see crackers)			
Grapefruit: Raw	1/2 (avg. size)	30	0.8
Grapes:			
White	20	75	1.0
Red or black	15-20	65	1.0
Green: (Snap) beans fresh or frozen	1/2 cup	10	2.1
Green peas: (see peas)			
Green peppers: (see peppers)			
Greens, cooked:			
Collards,			
Beet greens ,	1/2 cup	20	4.0
Dandelion, kale,			
Swiss chard			
Turnip greens	1/2 cup	20	4.0
Honeydew melon:	3" slice	42	1.5
Kasha: (see Buckwheat groats)			
Lasagna: (see Macaroni)			
Lentils:			
Brown, raw	1/3 cup	144	5.5
Brown, cooked	2/3 cup	144	5.5
Red, raw	1/2 cup	192	6.4
Red, cooked	1 cup	192	6.4
Lettuce: (Boston, leaf iceberg), shredded	1 cup	5	0.8
Macaroni:			
Whole wheat, cooked	1 cup	200	5.7
Regular, frozen with cheese, baked	10 oz	506	2.2
Muffins:			
English, whole wheat	1	125	3.7
Bran, whole wheat	1	136	4.6
Mushrooms:			
Raw	5 small	4	1.4
Sautéed or baked with 2 tsp diet margarine	4 large	45	2.0
Canned sliced, water-pack	1/4 cup	10	2.0
Noodles:			
Whole wheat egg	1 cup	200	5.7
Spinach whole wheat	1 cup	200	6.0
Okra: Fresh or frozen, cooked	1/2 cup	13	1.6
Olives:			
Green	6	42	1.2
Black	6	96	1.2
Onion:			
Raw	1 tbsp	4	0.2
Cooked	1/2 cup	22	1.5
Minced	1 tbsp	6	0.3
Green, raw (scallion)	1/4 cup	11	0.8
Orange:	1 large	70	2.4
	1 small	35	1.2

Food	Portion	Calories	Fiber (grams)
Parsley, chopped:	2 tbsp	4	0.6
	1 tbsp	2	0.3
Parsnip, pared, cooked:	1 large	76	2.8
	1 small	38	1.4
Peach:			
Raw	1 medium	38	2.3
Canned in light syrup	2 halves	70	1.4
Peanut Butter:			
Commercial	1 tbsp	86	1.1
Homemade	1 tbsp	70	1.5
Peanuts dry roasted:	1 tbsp	70	1.5
Pear:			
Raw	1 medium	88	4.0
Green, fresh or frozen	1/2 cup	60	9.1
Peas:			
Black-eyed: Frozen/canned	1/2 cup	74	8.0
Split peas, dried	1/2 cup	63	6.7
Split peas. cooked	1 cup	126	13.4
Peas and carrots frozen, 1/2 package	5 oz	40	6.2
Peppers:			
Green sweet raw	2 tbsp	4	0.3
Green sweet, cooked	1/2 cup	13	1.2
Red sweet (pimento)	2 tbsp	9	1.0
Red chili, fresh	1 tbsp	7	1.2
Dried, crushed	1 tsp	7	1.2
Pimento: (see Peppers)			
Pineapple:			
Fresh, cubed	1/2 cup	41	0.8
Canned	1 cup	58-74	0.8
Plums: Raw	2 or 3 small	38-45	2.0
Popcorn: (No oil, butter or margarine)	1 cup	20	1.0
Potatoes:			
Idaho, Baked	1 small (6 oz)	120	4.2
	1 med (7 oz)	140	5.0
All-purpose white/russet	1 small (60z)	60	2.2
Boiled 1 med	5 oz	100	3.5
Mashed (with 1 tbsp milk)	1/2 cup	85	3.0
Sweet baked or boiled (See also Yams)	1 small (5 oz)	146	4.0
Prunes pitted:	3	122	1.9
Radishes:	3	5	0.1
Raisins:	1 tbsp	29	1.0
Raspberries: Red fresh/frozen	1/2 cup	20	4.6
Raspberry jam:	1 tbsp	75	1.0
Rhubarb: cooked with sugar	1/2 cup	169	2.9
Rice:			
White (before cooking)	1/4 cup	150-190	1.0
Brown (before cooking)	1/4 cup	150-170	2.3
Instant	1/3 cup	170-190	1.0
Rutabaga: (yellow turnip)	1/2 cup	40	3.2
Sauerkraut: Canned	2/3 cup	15	3.1
Scallion: (see onion)			
Shredded wheat:			
Large biscuit	1 piece	74	2.2
Spoon size	1 cup	168	4.4
Spaghetti:			
Whole wheat, plain	1 cup	200	5.6
with meat sauce	1 cup	396	5.6
with tomato sauce	1 cup	220	6.0
Spinach:			
Raw	1 cup	8	3.5
Cooked	1/2 cup	26	7.0
Split peas: (See Peas)			

Food	Portion	Calories	Fiber (grams)
Squash:			
Summer (yellow)	1/2 cup	8	2.0
Squash winter, Baked or mashed	1/2 cup	40-50	3.5
Zucchini, raw or cooked	1/2 cup	7	3.0
Strawberries: Without sugar	1 cup	45	3.0
Succotash: (see corn)			
Sunflower: Kernels	1 tbsp	65	0.5
Sweet pickle relish:	1 tbsp	60	0.5
Sweet Potatoes: (see Potatoes)			
Swiss chard: (see Greens)			
Tomatoes:			
Raw	1 small	22	1.4
Canned	1/2 cup	21	1.0
Sauce	1/2 cup	20	0.5
Catsup	1 tbsp	18	0.2
Tortillas:			
White flour	large 8"	160	3.0
Cruz whole wheat	large 8"	130	11.0
La Tortilla Factory	large 8"	80	14.0
Mission low carb	6" size	110	11.0
Turnip:			
White raw, slivered	1/4 cup	8	1.2
Cooked	1/2 cup	16	2.0
Walnuts: English, Shelled, Chopped	1 tbsp	49	1.1
Watercress: Raw	1/2 cup	4	1.0
Watermelon:	1 thick slice	68	2.8
Wheat Thins: (see Crackers)			
Yams (orange fleshed sweet potato) cooked or baked in skin	1 med (6oz)	156	6.8

RESTING ENERGY CALCULATOR (REE)

Resting energy expenditure is equal to the number of calories required to maintain weight. All weight loss is dependent on one simple fact. To lose weight an individual must consume fewer calories than their calculated REE. REE can be calculated by the revised Harris-Benedict Equation. The revised Harris-Benedict Equation takes into account an individual's gender, height, weight and age. The REE can be calculated by inputting your height, weight and age in the appropriate equation. If you have access to the internet you may calculate your REE at the following website:

http://wwwusers.med.cornell.edu/~spon/picu/calc/beecalc.htm

Revised Harris-Benedict Equation

MALES
$66.5 + (6.25 \times lbs) + (12.7 \times inches) - (6.77 \times Age) = REE$

FEMALES
$665.1 + (4.34 \times lb) + (4.7 \times inches) - (4.676 \times Age) = REE$

REE is expressed in calories per day.
Height is expressed in inches.
Weight is expressed in pounds.
Age is expressed in years.

To lose weight an individual must decrease their caloric intake by multiplying their calculated REE x .8. Again, in order to lose weight your caloric intake must be lower than your REE. Therefore, if your calculated REE is 1200, you will not lose weight if you consume 1200 Calories. Weight loss will only occur if the caloric intake is decreased by 250 calories, or 1200 calories x .8. The North Star Diet and Weight Management System purposely does not contain a sub-1200 calorie diet as it often produces malnutrition in individuals unless followed precisely. We strongly recommend that if your calculated REE x .8 is less than 1200 calories you meet with a nutritionist or physician comfortable with weight-loss management to help you construct a safe caloric diet of fewer than 1200 calories.

Food Diary

Date_____

Breakfast   Calories

_____   _____
_____   _____
_____   _____
_____   _____
_____   _____

Snack

_____   _____
_____   _____

Lunch

_____   _____
_____   _____
_____   _____
_____   _____
_____   _____

Dinner

_____   _____
_____   _____
_____   _____
_____   _____
_____   _____

                    Daily Total   _____

Water/Diet soda (Pop)/Coffee/Tea (8-12) 8 oz servings a day

1)_____ 2)_____3)_____4)_____5)_____6)_____7)_____8)_____

9)_____10)_____11)_____12)_____

Name_____   EXERCISE LOG

Week of _____		
Day	Type of Exercise	Time
M		
Tu		
W		
Th		
F		
Sa		
Su		
	Total	

Week of _____		
Day	Type of Exercise	Time
M		
Tu		
W		
Th		
F		
Sa		
Su		
	Total	

Week of _____		
Day	Type of Exercise	Time
M		
Tu		
W		
Th		
F		
Sa		
Su		
	Total	

Week of _____		
Day	Type of Exercise	Time
M		
Tu		
W		
Th		
F		
Sa		
Su		
	Total	

Week of _____		
Day	Type of Exercise	Time
M		
Tu		
W		
Th		
F		
Sa		
Su		
	Total	

Week of _____		
Day	Type of Exercise	Time
M		
Tu		
W		
Th		
F		
Sa		
Su		
	Total	

Name_____   STEP EXERCISE LOG

Week of _____		
Day	Type of Exercise	Time
M		
Tu		
W		
Th		
F		
Sa		
Su		
	Total	

Week of _____		
Day	Type of Exercise	Time
M		
Tu		
W		
Th		
F		
Sa		
Su		
	Total	

Week of _____		
Day	Type of Exercise	Time
M		
Tu		
W		
Th		
F		
Sa		
Su		
	Total	

Week of _____		
Day	Type of Exercise	Time
M		
Tu		
W		
Th		
F		
Sa		
Su		
	Total	

Week of _____		
Day	Type of Exercise	Time
M		
Tu		
W		
Th		
F		
Sa		
Su		
	Total	

Week of _____		
Day	Type of Exercise	Time
M		
Tu		
W		
Th		
F		
Sa		
Su		
	Total	

Rules for the North Star Diet

1) Eat breakfast within 20 minutes after waking in the morning. Failure to eat a timely breakfast will decrease your fat-burning capacity, or metabolism. Breakfast choices consist of any high-fiber cereal with non-fat milk fortified with vitamin D and calcium or, preferably, non-fat soy milk fortified with vitamin D and calcium. High-fiber cereals should contain at least 8 grams of fiber in each serving. Recommended high-fiber cereals:

CEREAL	PORTION	CALORIES	FIBER (content)
General Mills Fiber One	1/2 cup	59	14 g
General Mills Fiber One Honey Clusters**	1 1/4 cup	170	14 g
Kellogg's Bran Buds	1/3 cup	80	11 g
Kellogg's All-Bran	1/2 cup	80	10 g
Post or Nabisco			
100% Bran	1/3 cup	80	9 g
Post Raisin Bran	1 cup	190	8 g
Kashi Good Friends	3/4 cup	90	8 g
Kashi Lean Crunch	1 cup	190	8 g
OATMEAL			
Quaker Weight Control	1 serving	160	8 g
TORTILLAS			
Cruz whole-wheat	large 8"	130	11 g
La tortilla factory	large 8"	80	14 g
Mission low carb	6" size	110	11 g

2) Consume mid-morning snacks and mid-afternoon snacks. Both snacks may consist of one (1200 calorie diet) or two (all other diets) of the following choices: banana; apple; pear; 2 cups strawberries (no sugar added); 1.5 cups blueberries (no sugar added); 2 cups raspberries (no sugar added); low-calorie yogurt (100 calories); 1 oz of soy nuts (100 calories total, varies based on brand and preparation); 1 oz soy chips (I recommend Revival brand soy chips). Failure to eat timely mid-morning and mid-afternoon snacks will decrease your fat-burning capacity, or metabolism. Three to four times a week you may substitute any food you desire(100 to 200 calories depending upon meal plan), for example one or two part-skim mozzarella cheese stick(s) or 1-2 oz of chocolate (100-200 calories).

Rules for the North Star Diet, cont'd.

3) Consume 2 liters of fluid a day (approximately 80 ounces). Eighty ounces of fluid is the equivalent of 8 ounces of water per hour for ten hours a day, or two 8-ounce glasses of water with each meal and snack. You may substitute diet soda pop or tea with meals if desired but no fruit juice or regular pop is allowed.

4) Consumption of two cups of green tea, one tea bag per cup, will promote 70 calories of weight loss on a daily basis. A personal favorite is Tazo Zen brand of green tea.

5) Consume dinner 3-4 hours prior to bed time. If you eat closer to bedtime there is an increased chance the food will be stored and converted into fat while you sleep. If you are still hungry after dinner, you may consume an apple, pear or banana or 1 ounce of lean, grilled protein, e.g. turkey, ham, beef, or fish.

6) The meal plans are to be used as guides. Most individuals only eat 7-10 different foods in a given week. If you like certain wraps or dinners and not others, consume those you enjoy the most. I only ask that starting in the second week of the North Star Diet you begin utilizing a whole-wheat wrap/tortilla. (See lunch alternative if you desire to use bread as an alternative). Whole-wheat wraps can often contain as much as 10 –14 g of fiber per serving. They are easy to make. Combine fillings in the center of the tortilla and roll up. I recommend the following whole-wheat tortilla/wraps: Cruz brand whole-wheat tortilla (10 grams of dietary fiber per serving); La Tortilla Factory whole-wheat, low-carb/low-fat tortillas (large size, 14 grams of fiber); and Carb Down flat bread (14 grams of fiber).

7) Consume daily: a multi-vitamin; 1200 mg of calcium carbonate; 1000 I.U. vitamin D; and 1000-3000 mg of fish oil.

** Personal Favorite

Day 1 Exercise Review

Exercise # 1

Exercise # 2

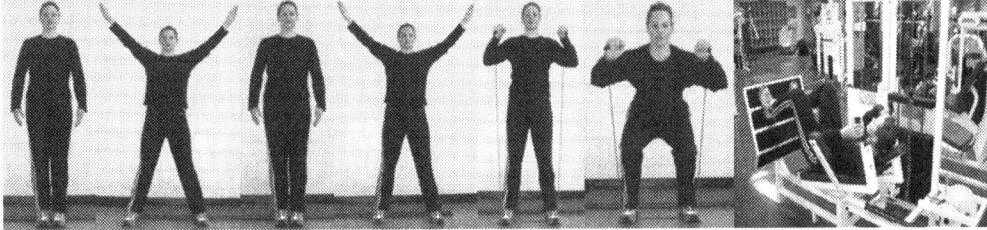

Fig 1   Fig 2   Fig 3   Fig 4   Fig 1   Fig 2   Fig 3

Exercise # 3

Exercise # 4

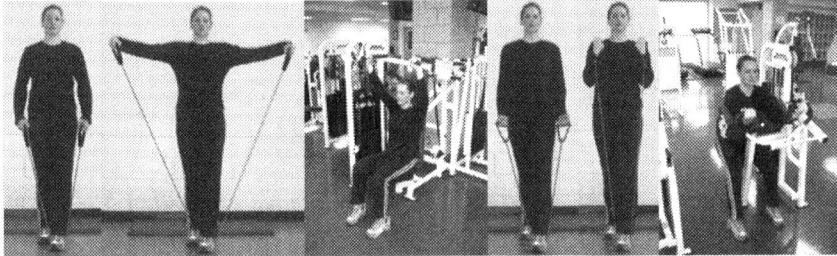

Fig 1   Fig 2   Fig 3   Fig 1   Fig 2   Fig 3

Exercise # 5

Exercise # 6

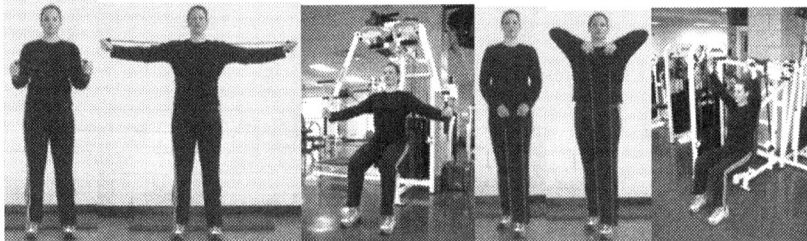

Fig 1   Fig 2   Fig 3   Fig 1   Fig 2   Fig 3

Exercise # 7

Exercise # 8

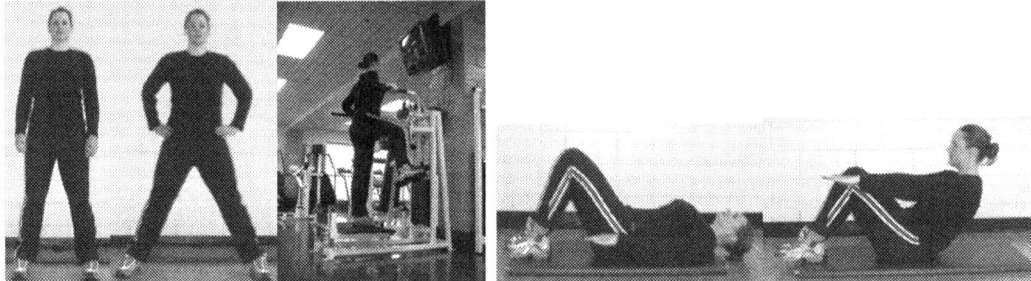

Fig 1   Fig 2   Fig 3   Fig 1   Fig 2

Day 2 Exercise Review

Exercise # 1

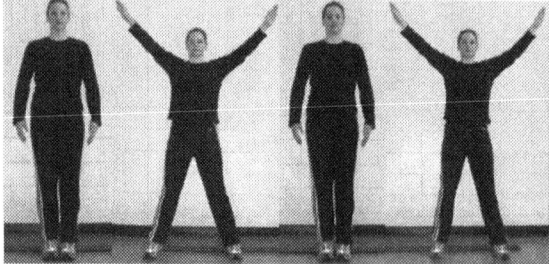

Fig 1   Fig 2   Fig 3   Fig 4

Exercise # 2

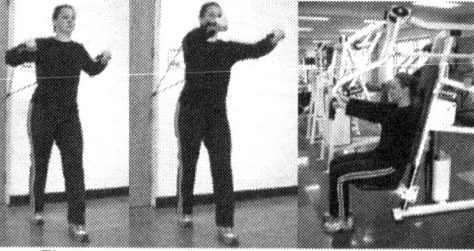

Fig 1   Fig 2   Fig 3

Exercise # 3

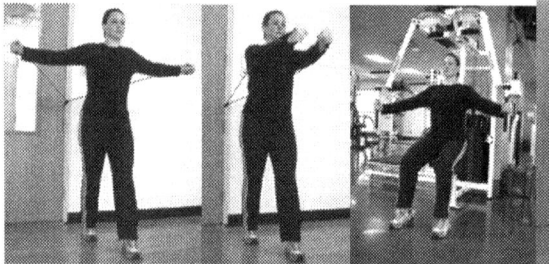

Fig 1   Fig 2   Fig 3

Exercise # 4

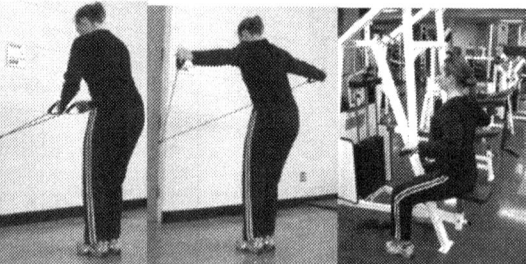

Fig 1   Fig 2   Fig 3

Exercise # 5

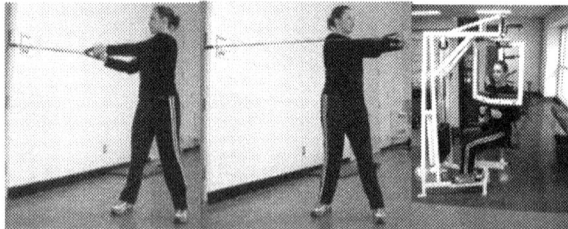

Fig 1   Fig 2   Fig 3

Exercise # 6

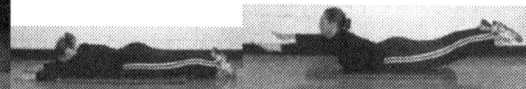

Fig 1   Fig 2

Exercise # 7

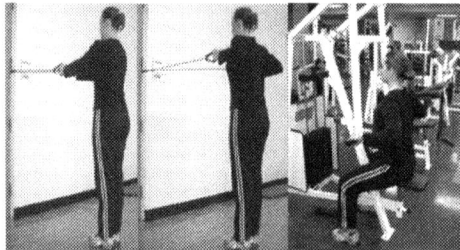

Fig 1   Fig 2   Fig 3

Exercise # 8

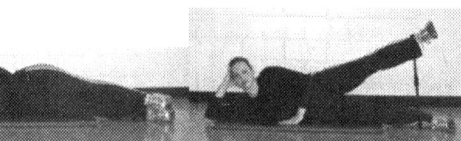

Fig 1   Fig 2

Day 3 Exercise Review

Exercise # 1

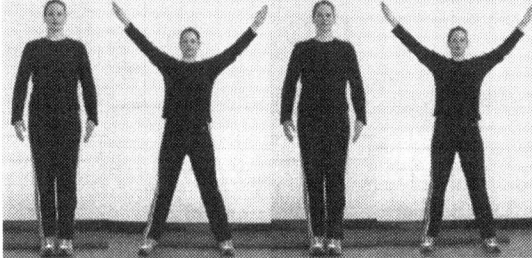

Fig 1   Fig 2   Fig 3   Fig 4

Exercise # 2

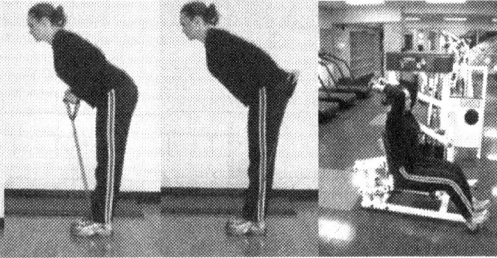

Fig 1   Fig 2   Fig 3

Exercise # 3

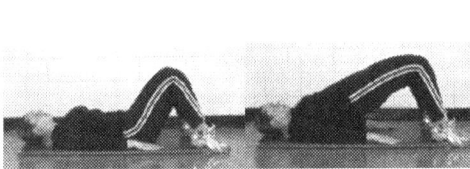

Fig 1   Fig 2

Exercise # 4

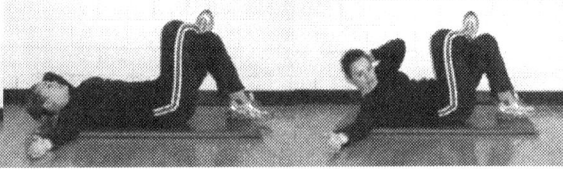

Fig 1   Fig 2

Exercise # 5

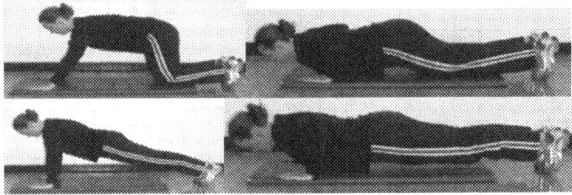

Fig 1   Fig 2

Exercise # 6

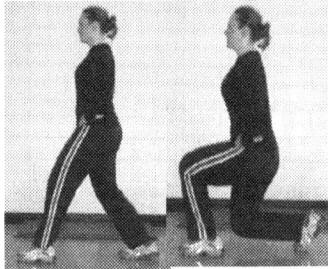

Fig 1   Fig 2

Exercise # 7

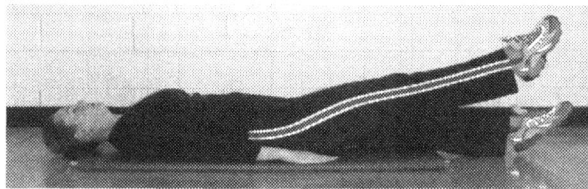

Exercise # 8

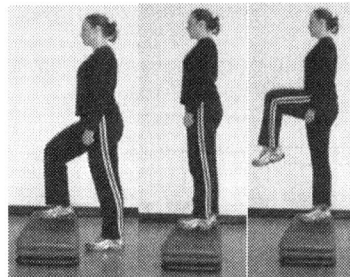

Fig 1   Fig 2   Fig 3

References:

Part One

Bravata DM, Sanders L, Huang J, et al. Efficacy and safety of low-carbohydrate diets: a systematic review. JAMA. 2003;289:1837-1850.

Samaha, FF, Iqbal N, Seshadri, P, et al. A low-carbohydrate as compared with a low-fat diet in severe obesity. N Engl J Med. 2003;348:2074-2081.

Sanders L. Big fat lies? The skinny on the low-carb high-fat diet. Special diets in weight management: do they work? Program and abstracts of the American College of Preventive Medicine 2004 Annual Meeting; February 18-22, 2002; Orlando, Florida. Session 33:55.

Part Two

Anderson JW. High-fiber diets for obese diabetic men on insulin therapy: short-term and long-term effects. In Vahouny GV, ed., Dietary fiber and obesity. Ne w York, Alan R. Liss. 1985;49-68.

Anderson JW, Sieling B. High fiber diets for obese diabetic patients. Obesity/ Bariatric Med 1980;9:109-113.

Booth DA. Food intake compensation for increase or decrease in the protein content of the diet. Behav Biol. 1974;12:31-40.

Brehm BJ, Seeley RJ, Daniels SR. A randomized trial comparing a very low carbohydrate diet and a calorie-restricted low fat diet on body weight and cardiovascular risk factors in healthy women. J Clin Endocrinol Metab. 2003;88:1617-1623.

Burley VJ, Blundell JE, Leeds AR. The effects of high and low fibre lunches on blood glucose, plasma insulin and hunger sensations. Int J Obes 1987;11(suppl 2):12.

Chih-Hsing Wu, Feng-Hwa Lu, Chin-Song Chang, Tsui-Chen Chang, Ru-Hsueh Wang and Chih-Jen Chang Relationship among Habitual Tea Consumption, Percent Bo dy Fat, and Body Fat Distribution Obesity Research 2003;11:1088-1095.

Crouse JR, 3rd, Morgan T, Terry JG, Ellis J, Vitolins M, Burke GL. A randomized trial comparing the effect of casein with that of soy protein containing varying amounts of isoflavones on plasma concentrations of lipids and lipoproteins. Arch Intern Med. 1999;159(17):2070-2076.

Dalais FS, Ebeling PR, Kotsopoulos D, McGrath BP, Teede HJ. The effects of soy protein containing isoflavones on lipids and indices of bone resorption in postmenopausal women. Clin Endocrinol (Oxf). 2003;58(6):704-709.

de Kleijn MJ, van der Schouw YT, Wilson PW, et al. Intake of dietary phytoestrogens is low in postmenopausal women in the United States: the Framingham study(1-4). J Nutr. 2001;131(6):1826-1832.

Divi RL, Chang HC, Doerge DR. Anti-thyroid isoflavones from soybean: isolation, characterization, and mechanisms of action. Biochem Pharmacol. 1997;54(10):1087-1096.

Doerge DR, Sheehan DM. Goitrogenic and es trogenic activity of soy isoflavones. Environ Health Perspect. 2002;110 Suppl 3:349-353.

Dulloo AG, Duret C, Rohrer D, Girardier L, Mensi N, Fathi M, Chantre P, and Vandermander J.
Efficacy of a green tea extract rich in catechin polyphenols and caffeine in increasing 24-h energy expenditure and fat oxidation in humans. Am. J. Clinic al Nutrition, Dec 1999; 70: 1040 - 1045.

Duncan K, Bacon JA, Weinsier RL. The effect of high and low energy density diets on satiety, energy intake, and eating time in obese and non-obese subjects . Am J Clin Nutr 1983;37:763-7.

Farshchi, H.R., Taylor, M.A., and Macdonald, I.A. (2204). Decreased thermic effect of food after an irregular compared with regular meal pattern in healthy lean women. International Journal of Obesity and Related Metabolic Disorders, 28, 653-660.

Goodman MT, Wilkens LR, Hankin JH, Lyu LC, Wu AH, Kolonel LN. Association of soy and fiber consumption with the risk of endometrial cancer. Am J Epidemiol. 1997;146(4):294-306.

Hill AJ, Blundell JE. Sensitivity of the appetite control system in obese subjects to nutritional and serotoninergic challenges. Int J Obes Relat Metab Disord. 1990;14:219-233.

Horn-Ross PL, John EM, Canchola AJ, Stewart SL, Lee MM. Phytoestrogen intake and endometrial cancer risk. J Natl Cancer Inst. 2003;95(15):1158-1164.
Howarth NC, Saltzman E, Roberts SB. Dietary fiber and weight regulation. Nutr Rev. 2001 May;59(5):129-39.

Jakicic JM, Wing RR: Strategies to improve exercise adherence: effect of short-bouts versus long-bouts of exercise. Med Science Spor ts Exerc 1997;29(5 suppl):S42

Jakicic JM, Winters C, Lang W, et al: Effects of intermittent exercise and use of home exercise equipment on adherence, weight loss, and fitness in overweight women: a randomized trial. JAMA 1999;282(16):1554-1560.

Jenkins DJ, Kendall CW, Jackson CJ, et al. Effects of high-and low-isoflavone soyfoods on blood lipids, oxidized LDL, homocysteine, and blood pressure in hyperlipidemic men and women. Am J Clin Nutr. 2002;76(2):365-372.

Jensen MK, Koh-Banerjee P, Hu FB, Franz M, Sampson L, Grønbæk M, and Rimm EB.
Intakes of whole grains, bran, and germ and the risk of coronary heart disease in men. Am. J. Clinical Nutrition, Dec 2004; 80: 1492 - 1499.

Knight EL, Stampfer MJ, Hankinson SE, Spiegelman D, Curhan GC. The impact of protein intake on renal function decline in women with normal renal function or mild renal insufficiency.
Ann Intern Med. 2003 Mar 18;138(6):460-7.

Landmesser U, Hornig B, Drexler H. Endothelial function: a critical determinant in atherosclerosis? Circulation. 2004;109(21 Suppl 1):II27-33.

Lichtenstein AH, Jalbert SM, Adlercreutz H, et al. Lipoprotein response to diets high in soy or animal protein with and without isoflavones in moderately hypercholesterolemic subjects. Arterioscler Thromb Vasc Biol. 2002;22(11):1852-1858.

Liu S, Willett WC, Manson JE, Hu FB, Rosner B, Colditz G. Relation between changes in intakes of dietary fiber and grain products and changes in weight and development of obesity among middle-aged women.
Am J Clin Nutr. 2003 Nov;78(5):920-7.

Ma, Y ., Bertone, E.R., Stanek, E.J. III, Reed, G.W., Hebert, J.R., Cohen, N.L., Merriam, P.A., Ockene, I.S. (2003). Association between eating patterns and obesity in a free-living us adult population. American Journal of Epidemiology.

Munro IC, Harwood M, Hlywka JJ, et al. Soy isoflavones: a safety review. Nutr Rev. 2003;61(1):1-33.

Nelson HD, Humphrey LL, Nygren P, Teutsch SM, Allan JD. Postmenopausal hormone replacement therapy: scientific review. JAMA. 2002;288(7):872-881.

Nuttall FQ. Gynecomastia as a physical finding in normal men. J Clin Endocrinol Metab. 1979 Feb;48(2):338-40.

Rolls BJ, Ello-Martin JA, Tohill BC. What can intervention studies tell us about the relationship between fruit and vegetable consumption and weight management? Nutr Rev. 2004 Jan;62(1):1-17.

Rolls BJ, Hetherington M, Burley VJ. The specificity of satiety: the influence of foods of different macronutrient content on the development of satiety. Physiol Behav. 1988;43:145-153.

Sagara M, Kanda T, M NJ, et al. Effects of dietary intake of soy protein and isoflavones on cardiovascular disease risk factors in high risk, middle-aged men in Scotland. J Am Coll Nutr. 2004;23(1):85-91.

Sanders TA, Dean TS, Grainger D, Miller GJ, Wiseman H. Moderate intakes of intact soy protein rich in isoflavones compared with ethanol-extracted soy protein increase HDL but do not influence transforming growth factor beta(1) concentrations and hemostatic risk factors for coronary heart disease in healthy subjects. Am J Clin Nutr. 2002;76(2):373-377.

Setchell KD, Lydeking-Olsen E. Dietary phytoestrogens and their effect on bone: evidence from in vitro and in vivo, human observational, and dietary intervention studies. Am J Clin Nutr. 2003;78(3 Suppl):593S-609S.

Stubbs RJ, van Wyk MC, Johnstone AM, Harbron CG. Breakfasts high in protein, fat or carbohydrate: effect on within-day appetite and energy balance. Eur J Clin Nutr. 1996;50:409-417.

Sunkin S, Garrow JS. The satiety value of protein. Hum Nutr Appl Nutr. 1982;36:197-201.

Tice JA, Ettinger B, Ensrud K, Wallace R, Blackwell T, Cummings SR. Phytoestrogen supplements for the treatment of hot flashes: the Isofla vone Clover Extract (ICE) Study: a randomized controlled trial. Jama. 2003;290(2):207-214.

Thomson CA, Rock CL, Giuliano AR, Newton TR, Cui H, Reid PM, Green TL, Alberts DS; Women's Healthy Eating & Living Study Group.Longitudinal changes in body weight and body composition among women previously treated for breast cancer consuming a high-vegetable, fruit and fiber, low-fat diet. Eur J Nutr. 2005 Feb;44(1):18-25. Epub 2004 Mar 5.

van Erp-Baart MA, Brants HA, Kiely M, et al. Isoflavone intake in four different European countries: the VENUS approach. Br J Nutr. 2003;89 Suppl 1:S25-30.

Washburn S, Burke GL, Morgan T, Anthony M. Effect of soy protein supplementation on serum lipoproteins, blood pressure, and menopausal symptoms in perimenopausal women. Menopause. 1999;6(1):7-13.

White LR, Petrovitch H, Ross GW, et al. Brain aging and midlife tofu consumption. J Am Coll Nutr. 2000;19(2):242-255.

Yao M, Roberts SB. Dietary energy density and weight regulation. Nutr Rev. 2001 Aug;59(8 Pt 1):247-58.

Zhang K, Sun M, Werner P, Kovera AJ, Albu J, Pi-Sunyer FX, Boozer CN.Sleeping metabolic rate in relation to body mass index and body composition. Int J Obes Relat Metab Disord. 2002 Mar;26(3):376-83.

Part Three

Dietary refernce intakes for energy, carbohydrate, fiber, fat, fatty acids, cholesterol, protein, and amino acids. National Academy Press 2002

Part Seven

Barascu A, Besson P, Le Floch O, Bougnoux P, Jourdan ML. CDK1-cyclin B1 mediates the inhibition of proliferation induced by omega-3 fatty acids in MDA-MB-231 breast cancer cells. Int J Biochem Cell Biol. 2005 Sep 26.

Boucher BJ. Inadequate vitamin D status: does it contribute to the disorders comprising syndrome 'X'? [published erratum appears in Br J Nutr 1998 Dec;80(6):585]. Br.J.Nutr. 1998;79:315-27.

Grant WB An ecologic study of dietary and solar ultraviolet-B links to breast carcinoma mortality rates.Cancer 2002 Jan 1;94(1):272-81.

Hansen CM, Binderup L, Hamberg KJ, Vitamin D and cancer: effects of 1,25(OH)2D3 and its analogs on growth control and tumorigenesis. Front Bios ci. 2001 Jul 1;6:D820-48.

Lamprecht SA, Lipkin M. Cellular mechanisms of calcium and vitamin D in the inhibition of colorectal carcinogenesis. Ann N Y Acad Sci. 2001 Dec;952:73-87.

Lane NE, Nevitt MC, Gore LR, Cummings SR. Serum levels of vitamin D and hip osteoarthritis in elderly women: a longitudinal study. Arthriti Rheum 1997; 40(suppl): S238.

Lieberman DA, Prindiville S, Weiss DG, Willett W. Risk Factors for Advanced Colonic Neoplasia and Hyperplastic Polyps in Asymptomatic Individuals. JAMA. 2003;290:2959-2967.

Luscombe CJ, French ME, Liu S, Prostate cancer risk: associations with ultraviolet radiation, tyrosinase and melanocortin-1 receptor genotypes.Br J Cancer. 2001 Nov;85(10):1504-9.

Majewski S, Kutner A, Jablonska S. Vitamin D analogs in cutaneous malignancies. Curr Pharm Des. 2000 May;6(7):829-38.

McAlindon TE, Felson DT, et al. Relation of dietary intake and serum levels of vitamin D to progression of osteoarthritis of the knee among participants in the Framingham Study. Ann Intern Med 1996; 125: 353-359

Mokady E, Schwartz B, Shany S, A protective role of dietary vitamin D3 in rat colon carcinogenesis. Nutr Cancer. 2000;38(1):65-73.

NHS Northern and Yorkshire Regional Drug And Therapeutics Center Drug Treatment OF Obesity. Wolfson Unit Claremont Place Newcastle upon Tyne NE2 4HH, July 1999.

Ortlepp JR, Lauscher J, Hoffmann R, The vitamin D receptor gene variant is associated with the prevalence of type 2 diabetes mellitus and coronary artery disease. Diabet Med. 2001 Oct;18(10):842-5.

Platz EA, Hankinson SE, Hollis BW, Plasma 1,25-dihydroxy- and 25-hydroxyvitamin D and adenomatous polyps of the distal colorectum.Cancer Epidemiol Biomarkers Prev. 2000 Oct;9(10):1059-65.

Tangpricha V, Flanagan JN, Whitlatch LW, 25-hydroxyvitamin D-1alpha-hydroxylase in normal and malignant colón tissue. Lancet. 2001 May 26;357(9269):1673-4.

Wortsman J, Matsuoka LY, Chen TC, Lu Z, Holick MF. Decreased bioavailability of vitamin D in obesity. Am J Clin Nutr. 2000 Sep;72(3):690-3.

Youngstedt SD, Kripke DF.Long sleep and mortality: rationale for sleep restriction. Sleep Med Rev. 2004 Jun;8(3):159-74.

Part Eight

Benezra LM, Nieman DC, Nieman CM, Melby C, Cureton K, Schmidt D, Howley ET, Costello C, Hill JO, Mault JR, Alexander H, Stewart DJ, Osterberg K. Intakes of most nutrients remain at acceptable levels during a weight management program using the food exchange system.
J Am Diet Assoc. 2001 May;101(5):554-61.

Benotti PN, Forse RA. The role of gastric surgery in the multidisciplinary management of severe obesity. Am J Surg 1995; 169: 361-7.

Kalarchian MA, Marcus MD, Wilson GT, Labouvie EW, Brolin RE, LaMarca LB.
Binge eating among gastric bypass patients at long-term follow-up.
Obes Surg. 2002 Apr;12(2):270-5.

NHS Northern and Yorkshire Regional Drug and Therapeutics Center Drug Treatment of Obesity. Wolfson Unit Claremont Place Newcastle upon Tyne NE2 4HH, July 1999.